Nursing
http://dx.doi.org/10.5772/intechopen.71632
Edited by Nilgun Ulutasdemir

Contributors

Vasfiye Bayram Değer, Nokuthula Sibiya, Frances Johnson, Mayumi Uno, Nilgun Ulutasdemir

Notice

Statements and opinions expressed in the chapters are these of the individual contributors and not necessarily those of the editors or publisher. No responsibility is accepted for the accuracy of information contained in the published chapters. The publisher assumes no responsibility for any damage or injury to persons or property arising out of the use of any materials, instructions, methods or ideas contained in the book.

First published in London, United Kingdom, 2018 by IntechOpen
IntechOpen is the global imprint of INTECHOPEN LIMITED, registered in England and Wales, registration number: 11086078, The Shard, 25th floor, 32 London Bridge Street
London, SE19SG – United Kingdom
Printed in Croatia

British Library Cataloguing-in-Publication Data
A catalogue record for this book is available from the British Library

Additional hard copies can be obtained from orders@intechopen.com

Nursing, Edited by Nilgun Ulutasdemir
p. cm.
Print ISBN 978-1-78923-775-7
Online ISBN 978-1-78923-776-4

NURSING

Edited by **Nilgun Ulutasdemir**

We are IntechOpen,
the world's leading publisher of
Open Access books
Built by scientists, for scientists

3,750+
Open access books available

115,000+
International authors and editors

119M+
Downloads

Our authors are among the

151
Countries delivered to

Top 1%
most cited scientists

12.2%
Contributors from top 500 universities

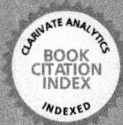

Interested in publishing with us?
Contact book.department@intechopen.com

Numbers displayed above are based on latest data collected.
For more information visit www.intechopen.com

Meet the editor

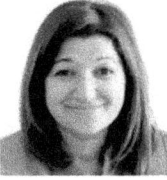

Nilgun Ulutasdemir graduated with a BSc degree from Hacettepe University in 1997, an MSc degree from Ankara University in 2004, and a PhD degree at the Fırat University, Faculty of Medicine, Department of Public Health in 2012. She became an assistant professor in 2012. She has been working at the University of Eurasia, Faculty of Health Sciences, since 2017. She is the head of the Department of Management and Administration of Health Facilities and assistant director of Health Science Institute. She has been assigned to scientific committees of several national and international conferences and has published several book chapters and papers in various countries. Her current research interests include public health, occupational health and safety, work stress, anxiety, first aid, elderly health, disabilities and cure, school health, and infectious diseases.

Contents

Preface

Nursing is one of the book titles proposed by InTech in 2017. I got very excited when I got the invitation to edit this book. It was a dream to collect various manuscripts from scientists throughout the world to discuss nursing in several countries. InTech's invitation made this dream come true. This book covers topics from nursing history and philosophy, communication and ethics in nursing, nursing, and culture. Thus, it can be used as a guide by student nurses and working nurses to recognize the nursing profession and to keep up with current developments.

In this book, you will find all aspects of nursing profession. To this extent, a wide array of nursing that includes nursing history, nursing philosophy, communication in nursing, ethics in nursing, and intercultural care has been discussed extensively.

The first step to cover was to select and disseminate the keywords, which helped us to receive numerous abstracts. These abstracts were then carefully evaluated, and those that were believed to contribute significantly to the literature were invited to take their place in this book. It took several months to edit each and every word of the sent chapters. It was a very fruitful feedback process that we had with our authors.

In this book, you will read chapters from authors in South Africa, Japan, USA and Turkey. They discussed the nursing issues from their perspectives and reflected and provided solution to the problems experienced from their own eyes. Thus, it makes the contents of this book interesting and very valuable.

I, hereby, would like to thank Ms. Anita Condic who helped me with positive attitude at every single step of the publication process.

Associate Professor Dr. Nilgun Ulutasdemir
University of Eurasia, Omer Yildiz Campus
Faculty of Health Sciences
Trabzon, Turkey

Introduction

Chapter 1

Introductory Chapter: Nursing

Nilgun Ulutasdemır

Additional information is available at the end of the chapter

http://dx.doi.org/10.5772/intechopen.79519

1. Introduction

Nursing is an applied health discipline dealing with the health conditions of the individual, family, and the community, which has succeeded in renewing and adapting itself to the daily social, cultural, and technological changes from the past to the present [1]. The Nurses' Day began to be celebrated since May 12, 1954 in honor of Florence Nightingale's birthday.

It has been defined by the International Nursing Council (ICN) as "a profession that helps to protect and improve the health of the individual, the family, and the community, and provides support for the rehabilitation and recovery from the diseases" [2]. The key role of nursing in health services was highlighted in all International Health Promotion Conferences, especially in Alma-Ata [3], followed by those in Ottawa [4] and Helsinki (2013) and also in the Commission Report of Social Determinants of World Health Organization. Increasing the role of nurses in public health services was also emphasized in international decisions about nursing especially by The European Nursing Conference-Vienna (1988), Munich Declaration (2000), and ICN reports (2008) [5–8].

Nursing is one of the leading professions that has an indispensable role in the protection and improvement of human health. The significance of the profession arises from the fact that the nurses work in a position where they help the most precious being in the world, i.e., individuals, in case of failure to meet basic needs themselves, protect and enable them to recover from illness, and so on. It is, therefore, imperative that nurses are trained thoroughly so that they are competent and capable enough to learn affective behaviors, cognitive, and technical skills in the provision of quality public nursing services [9].

Today, nurses have been able to perform functions fulfilled by professionals such as doing research, theory development, being member of professional organizations, and taking part in political activities, as well as providing health care [10]. Thus, the concepts of professionalism and professional values in nursing have come to the agenda. Nurses who have an important role in the provision of health services are among healthcare professionals [11].

The professional values that nurses have are guiding their interactions with healthy/sick individuals, colleagues, other team members, and the community as well as making decisions on value-added practices and providing the basis for nursing practice [12, 13].

In the past centuries when nursing was considered a female job, the similar evolution of the nursing profession to all other branches of science has allowed it to be regarded as a branch of science since the early twentieth century. Nursing, rooted in objective reality, and applying contemporary scientific knowledge to its own discipline, has increasingly begun to establish its own scientific generalizations and to produce its own theories. Nursing is considered as a science and art that is steadily developing every day and carrying out its applications with a rich content based on synthesis of both psychosocial interactions and biophysiological events [14].

Today, every aspect of life is undergoing a rapid and continuously changing process whose results are very closely related to individuals. Particularly, breakthroughs in medicine and technology contribute immeasurably to human health while leading to a more complex situation in areas where health care is provided. That is why nurses must constantly monitor changes and revolutions around the world and provide themselves with required skills and competences to deal with them [9].

Educators and administrators need to know, understand, and believe in the importance of intercultural nursing care in order to be role models for students. The first step in the development and implementation of intercultural nursing education programs in nursing institutions is to evaluate the curriculum. It is recommended that the review in nursing schools be started with an examination of the mission statement. It should be examined whether the significance of cultural differences, care, and education are explained in the mission statement [15, 16]. In terms of multiculturalism, important main subjects, concepts, and theories should be defined and integrated into the curriculum [16].

An educational environment should be created in which racial differences are accepted and respected in nursing education. Within the scope of the program, generalizations and conceptualizations specific to different cultural groups should be introduced in theoretical and practical courses. During the courses, social problems, experiences brought about by different racetracks such as racism, prejudicial discrimination, language problems, communicative difficulties, lack of obtaining information, health services that do not meet the needs, lack of recognition, or determination of diagnosis, and incorrect nursing diagnosis should be discussed [15–18].

This book covers topics from nursing history and philosophy, communication and ethic in nursing, evidence-based nursing, nursing, and culture. Thus, it can be used as a guide by student nurses and working nurses to recognize the nursing profession and to keep up with current developments. In this book, you will find all aspects of nursing profession. To this extent, a wide array of nursing that includes nursing history, nursing philosophy, communication in nursing, ethic in nursing, evidence-based care, and intercultural care has been discussed extensively.

Author details

Nilgun Ulutasdemır

Address all correspondence to: nulutasdemir@yahoo.com

Faculty of Health Science, Omer Yıldız Campus, University of Eurasia, Ortahisar, Trabzon, Turkey

References

[1] Akça Ay F. Basic professional concepts. In: Akça Ay F, editor. Basic Nursing Concepts, Principles, Applications. Istanbul: Istanbul Medical Publishing; 2010. p. 47

[2] International Counsel of Nursing (ICN). Available from: http://www.icn.ch/who-we-are/icn-definition-of-nursing/ [Accessed: April 28, 2018]

[3] World Health Organization (WHO). Declaration of Alma-ata: International Conference on Primary Health Care. 1978. Available from: http://www.who.int/hpr/NPH/docs/declaration_almaata.pdf [Accessed: April 28, 2018]

[4] World Health Organisation (WHO). Ottawa Charter for Health Promotion. Ottawa: Canadian Public Health Association. 1986. Available from: http://whqlibdoc.who.int/publications/1985/9241542020_eng.pdf [Accessed: April 28, 2018]

[5] Pektekin Ç. Nursing Philosophy: Theories, Care Models, Political Approaches. Istanbul: Istanbul Medical; 2011

[6] Reutter L, Kushner KE. Health equity through action on the social determinants of health: Taking up the challenge in nursing. Nursing Inquiry. 2010;**17**(3):269-280

[7] Smith M, Cusack L. The Ottawa charter-from nursing theory to practice: Insights from the area of alcohol and other drugs. International Journal of Nursing Practice. 2000;**6**(4):168-173

[8] World Health Organization (WHO). Commission on Social Determinants of Health-Final Report. Closing the gap in a generation: Health equity through action on the social determinants of health. Geneva, 2008. http://www.who.int/social_determinants/thecommission/finalreport/en/ [Access Date: 28 April 2018]

[9] https://www.medimagazin.com.tr/authors/gulten-uyer/tr-gecmisten-gelecege hemsirelik-cercevesinde-hemsirelige-vurgu-72-24-2506.html Emphasis on nursing in the context of nursing from the past to the future 06.09.2010 [Accessed: April 28, 2018]

[10] Karadag G, Ucan O. Nursing education and quality. Firat Health Services Journal. 2006;**1**:42-51

[11] Goris S, Kılıc Z, Ceyhan O, Senturk A. Nurses' professional values and affecting factors. Journal of Psychiatric Nursing. 2014;**5**(3):137-142

[12] Rassin M. Nurses' professional and personal values. Nurse Ethics. 2008;**15**:614-630

[13] Sellman D. Professional values and nursing. Medicine, Health Care, and Philosophy. 2011;**14**:203-208

[14] Bayık A. Nursing discipline and research: Principles and methods of research in nursing. In: Erefe I, editor. Association for Research and Development in Nursing-HEMAR-GE Publication. Vol. 1. Istanbul: Odak Offset; 2002. pp. 13-26

[15] Bayık Temel A. Intercultural (multicultural) nursing education. Atatürk University Nursing School Journal. 2008;**11**(2):92-101

[16] White HL. Implementing the multicultural education perspective into the nursing education curriculum. Journal of Instructional Psychology. 2003;**30**(4):326-332

[17] Narayanasamy A. Transcultural nursing: How do nurses respond to cultural needs? The British Journal of Nursing. 2003;**12**(2):36-45

[18] Nairn S, Hardy C, Paramal L, Williams GA. Multicultural or anti-racist teaching in nurse education: A critical appraisal. Nurse Education Today. 2004;**24**(3):188-195

Nursing History and Philosophy

Chapter 2

Choosing Your Philosophical Slat

Frances Mary Johnson

Additional information is available at the end of the chapter

http://dx.doi.org/10.5772/intechopen.74919

Abstract

The development of nursing knowledge and history of nursing as a profession began with Florence Nightingale who served in the Crimean War by caring for the wounded in Scutari and her establishment of a School of Nursing at St. Thomas hospital in London. Nursing has since continued to evolve to its twenty-first-century focus, which entails sophisticated nursing theories that are utilized to guide research, practice, education, and administration. This chapter serves as an introduction to the nursing student and focuses on the definition of a nursing metaparadigm and its concepts. It briefly touches upon the history and growth of nursing as a profession since its inception. It gives the beginner nursing student an explanation of nursing theory and its separate subcomponents. It describes the relationship between nursing theory, practice, and research. Instructions are put forth as to how to formulate a research question. It gives a brief explanation of the different types of research design. The overall goal of the chapter is to assist the novice student to gain practical knowledge to begin a research study.

Keywords: philosophy, research practice/theory, philosophical focus

1. Introduction

The goal of this chapter is to gain an understanding of the basic nursing concepts which will enable the nursing student to formulate a research question. It begins with the discussion of the definition of the nursing metaparadigm and its components. It briefly describes the evolution of nursing knowledge and includes the state of nursing science as it exists in the United States. This is followed by a description of nursing models and theories and includes examples to illustrate the different levels of nursing theory development. This is followed by a brief introduction depicting the relationship between nursing theory and practice. The basic types of research are described, as well as practical tips for formulating a nursing research question. An introduction referencing the influence of Western nursing scholars in other parts of the world is described. Tips for interdisciplinary collaboration amongst researchers with like interests and goals are put forth.

2. The nursing metaparadigm

The central themes and unifying concepts that form the basis of nursing in their broadest sense constitute the nursing metaparadigm. Traditionally speaking the four concepts inherent in the nursing metaparadigm are person, environment, health, and nursing [1]. The metaparadigm forms the backbone, figuratively speaking, of what it is that we as nurses do. These metaparadigm concepts are tied together by the laws that govern the highest function of the health of a human being, how the human being interfaces with the environment, and the process by which positive or negative changes in health ensue [1].

A person is defined as the one receiving the nursing care. Environment is viewed as the area or space wherein the person exists. Health is seen as the point where the patient is along the health-illness continuum. Nursing is the action taken by the nurse [2]. A nursing theorist defines each of these metaparadigm concepts in accordance with their worldview of nursing. Thus a metaparadigm can be thought of as an overarching principle or umbrella covering our outlook that defines our practice.

As a nurse, it is important to take an inventory of ourselves by examining how we were brought up, what we assume to be true, what beliefs we hold dear, and what our values entail. This will assist us in defining our worldview that guides and influences our practice. This can be done by examining our cultural beliefs, how we were raised as a child, parental relationships, era in which we were part of, social views, as well as any other influences that have had a major impact on our lives. Assumptions, beliefs, and values guide our practice. It is through the process of self-inventory and self-realization that one can identify their own unique worldview. It is equally important for a nurse to be able to understand the worldviews of the patients whom we serve. This enables us to convey understanding and compassion in our interactions, which ultimately promotes health and healing.

The study of how nurse scientists define metaparadigm concepts defines our profession.

As related to paradigms, Kuhn states, "By studying the and by practicing with them, the members of their corresponding community learn their trade" ([3], p. 43).

To illustrate, holism is a concept that is used in the nursing arena to define the metaparadigm concept of person. Embodiment is a unique state that refers to how patients experience themselves. Nursing is beginning to see that the understanding of patient embodiment is central to providing patient care. The author proposes that nursing is evolving to include the understanding of both the patient and the nurse embodiment as central to care for a patient. It is proposed that nurses face a challenge of reflecting on their own embodiment and whether their persona interferes with the practice of providing holistic care [4]. This implies the importance of self-knowledge as well as cultural sensitivity as a basis for holistic care.

3. History of the nursing knowledge

The history of nursing as a profession began with Florence Nightingale who served in the Crimean War by caring for the wounded in Scutari and her establishment of a School of Nursing at St. Thomas hospital in London. The 1900s–1940s marked the curriculum era in nursing. During this time emphasis was placed on the curriculum content needed to train nurses. The 1950s–1970s focused on the role for nurses and content for nursing research. This era also formulated the role and program content for the advanced nursing role and graduate education. The 1980s–1990s focused on nursing theory or how one looks at the way in which theories guide research and practice. Nursing in the twenty-first century focuses on the way in which nursing theories are utilized and how nursing theory guides research, practice, education, and administration [5].

4. What is nursing theory?

A nursing theory is "a creative and rigorous structuring of ideas that projects a tentative purposeful, and systematic view of a phenomenon" ([6], p. 106). A nursing theory contains concepts, definitions, relationships, and assumptions derived from models. The purpose is to describe, gain understanding, predict, and/or prescribe what will take place in phenomenon. The researcher uses either deductive or inductive reasoning to derive a theory [7]. Concepts are a part of a phenomenon and as such are abstract. Constructs on the other hand consist of groups of concepts. For example, patient-centered care is a construct. It can consist of many concepts which can include participation, respect, and collaboration. Theories can be formulated which center around assumptions referencing these concepts.

A *grand theory* is a type of theory that was originated by C.W. Mills. It is viewed as an abstract formal organization of concepts that are used to view and take precedence over the social world [8]. For example, complexity science is a twenty-first-century worldview that views the world as systems that are complex and interact in a dynamic interactive fashion which is unpredictable. It is not a single theory but a guiding framework. A key concept to complexity theory is the complex adaptive system (CAS). A CAS is a group of individual components that are interconnected in such a manner that the action of one changes that context of another. Families or committees are two examples. Systems have fuzzy boundaries, and this can lead to challenges in problem solving [8]. For example, suppose a day-care facility decided to change their hours from 0700 to 1900 to 0800–1600, one can realize the havoc that this would cause on family members that have set work hours, child routines, family and day-care budgets, and employers. Some of the other tenets of CAS are that agents respond to their environment by using an internalized set of rules and that these rules determine the agent's actions. The agents in the system are adaptive and the systems are intertwined or embedded within other systems and evolve interdependently [9].

Middle-range theories were proposed by R.K. Merton. They consist of hypothesis that can be tested. They are made up of propositions and though abstract are derived from grand theories. They are close enough to everyday observable data to be incorporated into a set of propositions [10]. They form the basis for clinical research and can be applied to multiple settings. For example, concepts such as *pain, stress, and comfort* have been instrumental in defining a theoretical basis for nursing practice through the use of middle-range theories early in the evolution of nursing.

Nursing models differ from nursing theories in that a model provides us with a structure whereas a theory is a set of ideas.

A case can be made such that consideration is given to the use of grand theories as a context for their work due to the complexity of patient-care issues. An example is cited referencing the impact of conditions such as HIV-AIDS and the impact not only on the client but the family, community, nation, and the world. Neuman's systems model was referenced as a good choice [11].

5. The connection between nursing theory practice and research

Research ignites nursing knowledge. The structure of nursing knowledge is composed of metaparadigm concepts, philosophical positions, conceptual models, nursing theories, and nursing indicators [12]. These structural components guide research which helps in further defining practice. Implementation of evidence-based practice serves as the impetus for further research thereby refining our nursing scientific basis for practice. Nursing philosophy is "a statement of foundational and universal assumptions, beliefs, and principles about the nature of knowledge and thought (epistemology) and about the nature of the entities represented in the metaparadigm (i.e., nursing practice and human health processes [ontology])" ([13], p. 76).

6. Developing nursing knowledge

Using a theory to guide a research study guides the researcher in formulating the research question, hypothesis/hypotheses that are being tested, and guides the researcher in interpreting the results. The first step in formulating a research question is determining the area of interest and a tentative focus for a study question. Once the focus is identified, it is best to go to the literature to see what has been studied, what literature gaps exist, and how you can formulate a research study that will both assist you in your clinical inquiry and be of most benefit to the profession. It is also important to identify a theory that reflects your own beliefs, values, and philosophy. It is equally important to identify a theory that naturally lends itself to guiding the study. The PICOT method is a concise method utilized to formulate a research question. (P)—Population refers to the sample of subjects that you will gather for your study. (I)—Intervention refers to the treatment that is the focus of the study. (C)—Comparison refers to the reference group that you will compare to your treatment group. (O)—refers to how you plan on measuring the effectiveness of your intervention. (T)—Time refers to the time period duration for your data collection [14].

Once your research topic's philosophical focus and framework are identified, the next step is to determine what type of design suits your study. In general, there are three broad types of research designs. These are qualitative, quantitative, and mixed methods. Quantitative research is often termed "experimental research." It uses statistics to measure results. Qualitative research on the other hand is a form of research used to explain people's beliefs, attitudes, and behaviors that occur in a social setting. The data that is obtained is nonnumeric. The mixed method approach utilizes a combination of qualitative and quantitative research. Some of the subtypes of quantitative include the experimental, correlational, or survey approach. The aim of experimental research is to determine cause and effect. Correlational research does not seek to find causation but correlations or associations. Survey research involves the administration of a questionnaire to a group of people. General types of qualitative research can include but are not limited to grounded theory, ethnographic, and narrative research. Grounded theory research is the study of a concept. It allows you to develop a theory concerning the concept. Ethnographic research is the study of people and cultures. Narrative research focuses on the lives of people, as they tell their own story.

Factors to consider in choosing your method of study can include what you want to study, your time limits, availability of your study sample, institutional requirements, and results of your literature search. These factors as aforementioned must be incorporated in a well-fitting philosophical focus and framework. It is in this way that your findings once incorporated into practice can generate further research.

7. Cross-country development of nursing knowledge

The development of nursing theory and knowledge development in other countries has been influenced by the United States. For example, nursing theory, its relationship to knowledge development, and scholarship in Iceland is 50 years old. University-based nursing education was established at the University of Iceland in 1973. This was the first baccalaureate nursing program in Europe. Nursing concepts such as holism, caring, adaptation, patient respect/partnerships, therapeutic relationships, and education as derived from Nightingale, Henderson, Peplau, and Roy influenced this curriculum. The introduction of some nursing theories, particularly Henderson's needs-based theory, along with United States nursing scholars such as Benner, Newman, Orem, and Parse, were cited as major influences in guiding practice [15].

China experienced a 30-year abolition of nursing academia from 1953 to 1983. United States' influence on nursing curriculum became apparent in 2001. Textbooks included information on US nursing theorists such as Henderson, Orem, Peplau, Rogers, and King. Prior to this the curriculum was medically focused and nurses were taught by physicians, due to lack of nursing faculty [16].

Nursing practice and education in Australia originated from the British tradition influenced by Florence Nightingale. The focus was on the medical model of care until the late 1960s. Henderson's nursing perspective influenced practice in the 1970s. Though Western nursing theory was taught in the schools, Australian nursing leaders cautioned against importing these theories on the premise that nursing being a practice discipline and influenced by contextual factors is most appropriately developed through the study of nursing practice in context [17].

Nevertheless, health for all and shared resources has been a goal of the World Health Organization (WHO) since the 1970s. The question arises as to how we as nurses can aspire to this goal. Though implementation of nursing interventions may present more of a challenge in different areas of the world, due to such factors as lack of resources and different government infrastructures, inter-disciplinary collaboration can be a means to troubleshoot the different challenges that arise. After the area of research is defined, it is suggested that the novice nurse seeks mentors that have like research interests and if possible from other areas of the world. In choosing a mentor, it would be important that the novice nurse not only chooses a colleague with the same interest but with a similar nursing philosophy and worldview. If the topic is new and unexplored, qualitative research may be a good place to start. If the literature review reveals a fair amount of studies with standardized tools and metrics, quantitative research may be the likely choice. Social media, blogs, Skype, and teleconferences are useful tools for developing intercollaborative research studies. Differences in outcomes can not only inspire new research to gain further understanding but also add further insight into the growing body of knowledge that is being developed.

8. Conclusion

In summary, the definition of a nursing metaparadigm and its related concepts has been reviewed. The history and growth of nursing as a profession has been briefly described. The relationship between nursing theory, practice, and research has been proposed. Pointers have been suggested to assist the student in the formulation of a research question. The chapter concludes with a brief explanation of the different types of research design and tips for assisting the novice student to gain practical knowledge to begin a research study and launch their new career.

Recommendations

It is recommended that the novice nurse take a self-inventory to define their unique world view of nursing. Once this is defined, a research interest for study needs to be identified. This is followed by an extensive literature search. During this time it is important to identify a theoretical framework which can guide your research. It is also important to identify potential mentors that will guide you along the way. Once gaps in the literature are identified, the next step is to develop the research question and method. It is important to network with colleagues with like interests to develop intercollaborative partnerships so that collectively we as nurses can further the WHO goal of health for all and shared resources.

Acknowledgments

Frances Mary Johnson, PhD, ANP-BC, AOCN, CNS currently works for the Department of Defense, Carl R. Darnall Army Medical Center in Fort Hood, Texas, as an Oncology Nurse

Practitioner. She has received her undergraduate nursing degree from Fairfield University in Fairfield, Connecticut, and MSN from Boston University in medical surgical nursing with an oncology focus in the CNS tract. She later received her nurse practitioner certificate from the University of Texas with a dual certification in adult health and oncology. She received her PhD from Texas Woman's University. Her experience includes extensive clinical care in both the oncology and primary care settings and extensive work in writing oncology programs standards. Her research interest is Oncology Nurse Practitioner Patient Navigation. She has published several articles and written and co-authored a book chapter on this topic. Her pastimes include piano, yoga, writing, hiking, and pet care.

Conflict of interest

There are no conflicts of interest.

Author details

Frances Mary Johnson

Address all correspondence to: roseypumpkin@mail.com

Department of Defense, Carl R. Darnall Army Medical Center in Fort Hood, Texas, USA

References

[1] Fawcett J. The metaparadigm of nursing: Present status and future refinements. The Journal of Nursing Scholarship. 1984;**16**(3):84-87

[2] Flaskerud J, Halloran E. Areas of agreement in nursing theory development. Advances in Nursing Science. 1980;**3**(1):1-7

[3] Kuhn T. The Structure of Scientific Revolutions. Chicago: University of Chicago Press; 1970

[4] Mason D. Holism and embodiment in nursing using Goethean science to join 2 perspectives on patient care. Holistic Nursing Practice. 2014;**28**(1);55-64. DOI: 10.1097/HNP. 0000000000000010

[5] Alligood M. Nursing Theory Utilization and Application. St. Louis: Elsevier; 2014

[6] Chin P, Kramer M. Theory and Nursing. St Louis: Mosby; 1995

[7] Current Nursing.com. Nursing Theories. Available from: http://currentnursing.com/ nursing_theory/nursing_theories_overview.html [Accessed: Feb 4, 2012]

[8] Mills C. The Sociological Imagination. New York: Oxford University Press; 1959

[9] Plsek P, Greenhalgh T. The challenge of complexity in health care. British Medical Journal. 2001;**323**(7313):625-628

[10] Merton R. Social Theory and Social Structure. Enlarged ed. New York: The Free press; 1968

[11] Florczak K, Poradzisz M, Hampson S. Nursing in a complex world. Nursing Science Quarterly. 2012;**25**(4):307-312. DOI: 10. 1177/0894318412457069

[12] Fawcett J, Desanto-Madeya S. Contemporary Nursing Knowledge: Analysis and Evaluation of Nursing Models and Theories. Philadelphia: F.A. Davis Company; 2013

[13] Reed P. A treatise on nursing knowledge development for the 21st century. Advances in Nursing Science. 1995;**17**(3):70-84

[14] Guyatt G, Drummond R, Meade M, Cook D. The Evidence-based Medicine Working Group. Users' Guides to the Medical Literature. 2nd ed. Chicago: McGraw Hill; 2008

[15] Jonsdottir H. Nursing theories and their relationship to knowledge development in Iceland. Nursing Science Quarterly. 2001;**14**(2):165-168

[16] Xu Y, Xu Z, Zhang J. A comparison of nursing education curriculum in China and the United States. Journal of Nursing Education. 2002;**41**(7):310-316

[17] Daly J, Jackson D. On the use of nursing theory in nurse education, nursing practice, and nursing research in Australia. Nursing Science Quarterly. 1999;**12**(4):342-345

Communication and Ethic in Nursing

Chapter 3

Effective Communication in Nursing

Maureen Nokuthula Sibiya

Additional information is available at the end of the chapter

http://dx.doi.org/10.5772/intechopen.74995

Abstract

Nurses are critical in the delivery of essential health services and are core in strengthening the health system. They bring people-centred care closer to the communities where they are needed most, thereby helping improve health outcomes and the overall cost-effectiveness of services. Nurses usually act as first responders to complex humanitarian crises and disasters; protectors and advocates for the community and communicators and co-ordinators within teams. Communication is a core component of sound relationships, collaboration and co-operation, which in turn are essential aspects of professional practice. The quality of communication in interactions between nurses and patients has a major influence on patient outcomes. Increases in nursing communication can lessen medical errors and make a difference in positive patient outcomes. This chapter explores how effective communication and interpersonal skills can enhance professional nursing practice and nursing relationships with various stakeholders. It explains principles of communication, communication process, purpose of communication, types of communication, barriers to effective communication, models of communication and strategies of improving communication and guidelines for successful therapeutic interactions.

Keywords: communication, communication skills, feedback, non-verbal communication, nurse–patient relationship, nursing verbal communication

1. Introduction

Nurses are critical in the delivery of essential health services and are core in strengthening the health system [1, 2]. They bring people-centred care closer to the communities where they are needed most, thereby helping improve health outcomes and the overall cost-effectiveness of services [3]. Nurses usually act as first responders to complex humanitarian crises and disasters; protectors and advocates for the community and communicators and co-ordinators within teams. Communication skills for nurses are essential but may be difficult to master.

Communication is the exchange of information between people by sending and receiving it through speaking, writing or by using any other medium. Clear communication means that information is conveyed effectively between people. To be a successful nurse, excellent communication skills are required [4]. Nurses speak to people of varying educational, cultural and social backgrounds and must do so in an effective, caring and professional manner, especially when communicating with patients and their families [5]. The quality of communication in interactions between nurses and patients has a major influence on patient outcomes. This influence can play a very important role in areas such as patient health, education and adherence [6]. Good communication plays an important role in the organization's effective functioning [7–9]. A nurse must therefore, continuously try to improve his/her communication skills as poor communication can be dangerous and lead to confusion.

2. Principles of communication

Principles of communication can be summarized as follows:

- Communication is a process;
- Communication is not linear, but circular;
- Communication is complex;
- Communication is irreversible; and
- Communication involves the total personality [5].

3. Communication process

Interaction between people is cyclic, which means that what one person says and does evokes a reaction from the other person, and this reaction again stimulates another reaction from the first person [10, 11]. Three things are needed for successful communication. They are:

1. A sender;
2. A clear message; and
3. A receiver [12].

4. Purpose of communication

The purpose of communication is to inquire, inform, persuade, entertain, request and investigate. A single message can have one or more of the following purposes:

- To convey information/opinion, for example, "I have headache" or "I am here to give you medication".

- To request information/opinion/behavior, for example, "Are you allergic to penicillin?" or "Tell me more about the injury".

- To give social acknowledgement, for example, "Hello" or "Good morning".

These three primary types of messages can be combined in many ways so that they form an interaction (conversation). The goals of the interaction can be comprehensive. Nurses strive to make all their communication with patients therapeutic, that is, their communication is purposefully and consciously planned to promote the patient's health and wellbeing.

5. Types of communication

Verbal and non-verbal communications are the two main types of communication used by human beings.

5.1. Verbal communication

Verbal communication is associated with spoken words and is vitally important in the health-care context. Members of the multi-disciplinary healthcare team communicate verbally with one another and with patients as well as family members.

5.2. Verbal communication

Non-verbal communication is not reliant on words. It is sent through the use of one's body rather than through speech or writing. This kind of communication, called body language, can tell a great deal or can totally the wrong impression. It is worth noting that body language may indicate a different meaning to what is spoken. As approximately 60% of communication is non-verbal, non-verbal skills are essential for effective communication [8]. Often non-verbal messages send stronger signals than verbal messages. Non-verbal communication is made up of:

- Accent

- Bodily contact

- Direction of gaze

- Emotive tone in speech

- Facial and gestural movements

- Physical appearance

- Posture

- Proximity

- Speech errors

- Timing of speech [5, 8–10].

6. Communication process

The communication process may be explained by means of a linear model of communication, interactive model of communication or transactional model of communication [11].

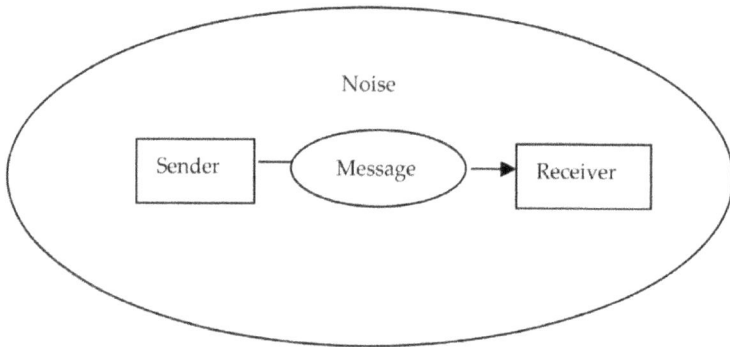

Figure 1. Linear model of communication.

6.1. Linear model of communication

Linear model of communication entails a sender, a message, a receiver and noise (**Figure 1**).

6.2. Interactive model of communication

Interactive model of communication gives a slightly more complex explanation of the communication process. Communication is seen as a process in which the listener gives feedback or responds to a message after a process of interpretation. A communicator creates and interprets a message with a personal field of expertise and/or a frame of reference **Figure 2**).

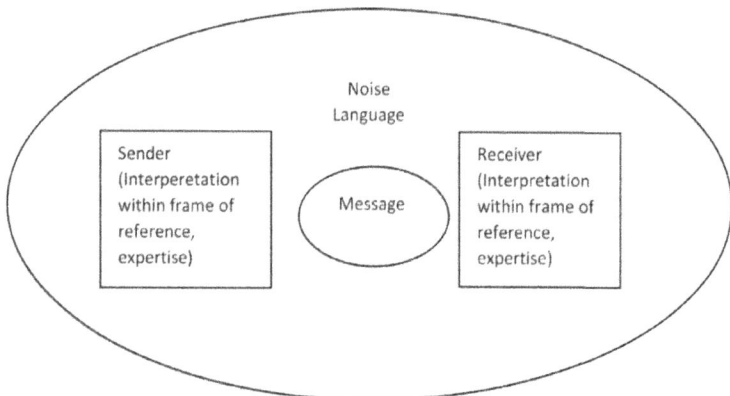

Figure 2. Interactive model of communication.

6.3. Transactional model of communication

Transactional model of communication acknowledges and gives emphasis to the dynamic nature of interpersonal communication and the multiple roles of the communicators. Features such as time, messages, noise, fields of experience, frames of reference, meanings, shared systems of communicators and personal systems all pay a role in the process of communication. Communicators often participate simultaneously (sending, receiving and interpreting). The unique interpretive and perceptual processes of individuals thus play an essential role in the communication process.

7. Barriers to effective communication

Effective communication skills and strategies are important for nurses. Clear communication means that information is conveyed effectively between the nurse, patients, family members and colleagues. However, it is recognized that such skills are not always evident and nurses do not always communicate well with patients, family members and colleagues. The message sent may not be the message received. The meaning of a message depends on its literal meaning, the non-verbal indicators accompanying it and the context in which it is delivered. It is therefore, easy to misinterpret the message, or to interpret it correctly, but to decide not to pursue its hidden meaning this leads to obstruction to communication. Continuous barriers to effective communication brings about a gradual breakdown in relationships. The barriers to effective communication outlined below will help nurses to understand the challenges [8].

7.1. Language barrier

Language differences between the patient and the nurse are another preventive factor in effective communication. When the nurse and the patient do not share a common language, interaction between them is strained and very limited [9–11]. Consequently, a patient may fail to understand the instructions from a nurse regarding the frequency of taking medication at home.

7.2. Cultural differences

Culture is another hindrance. The patient's culture may block effective nurse–patient interactions because perceptions on health and death are different between patients [12–14]. The nurse needs to be sensitive when dealing with a patient from a different culture [9, 15, 16]. What is acceptable for one patient may not be acceptable for another. Given the complexity of culture, no one can possibly know the health beliefs and practices of every culture. The nurse needs check with the patient whether he/she prefers to be addressed by first name or surname. The use of eye contact, touching and personal space is different in various cultures and rules about eye contact are usually complex, varying according to race, social status and gender. Physical contact between sexes is strictly forbidden in some cultures and can include handshakes, hugging or placing a hand on the arm or shoulder. A 'yes' does not always mean 'yes'. A smile does not indicate happiness, recognition or agreement. Whenever people communicate, there is a tendency to make value judgements regarding those perceived as being different. Past experiences can change the meaning of the message. Culture, background and bias can be good if they allow one to use past experiences to understand something new; it is when they change meaning of the message that they interfere with the communication process [12]. It is important for nurses to think about their own experiences when considering cultural differences in communication and how these can challenge health professionals and service users.

7.3. Conflict

Conflict is a common effect of two or more parties not sharing common ground. Conflict can be healthy in that it offers alternative views and values. However, it becomes a barrier to communication when the emotional 'noise' detracts from the task or purpose. Nurses aim for collaborative relationships with patients, families and colleagues.

7.4. Setting in which care is provided

The factors in care setting may lead to reduction in quality of nurse–patient communication. Increased workload and time constraints restrict nurses from discussing their patients concerns effectively [16]. Nurses work in busy environments where they are expected to complete a specific amount of work in a day and work with a variety of other professionals, patients and their families. The roles are hard, challenging and tiring. There is a culture to get the work done. Some nurses may consider colleagues who spend time talking with patients to be avowing the 'real' work and lazy. Nurses who might have been confident in spending time with patients in an area where this was valued, when faced with a task-orientated culture have the dilemma of fitting into the group or being outside the group and spending time engaging with patients. Lack of collaboration between the nurses and the doctors in information sharing also hinder effective communication. This leads to inconsistencies in the information given to patients making comprehension difficult for the patient and their families.

7.5. Internal noise, mental/emotional distress

Internal noise has an impact on the communication process. Fear and anxiety can affect the person's ability to listen to what the nurse is saying. People with feelings of fear and anger can find it difficult to hear. Illness and distress can alter a person's thought processes. Reducing the cause of anxiety, distress, and anger would be the first step to improving communication.

7.6. Perception

If a healthcare professional feels that the person is talking too fast, not fluently, or does not articulate clearly etc., he/she may dismiss the person. Our preconceived attitudes affect our ability to listen. People tend to listen uncritically to people of high status and dismiss those of low status.

7.7. Difficulty with speech and hearing

People can experience difficulty in speech and hearing following conditions like stroke or brain injury. Stroke or trauma may affect brain areas that normally enable the individual to comprehend and produce speech, or the physiology that produces sound. These will present barriers to effective communication.

7.8. Medication

Medication can have a significant effect on communication for example it may cause dry mouth or excess salivation, nausea and indigestion, all of which influence the person's ability and motivation to engage in conversation. If patients are embarrassed or concerned that they will not be able to speak properly or control their mouth, they could be reluctant to speak.

7.9. Noise

Equipment or environmental noise impedes clear communication. The sender and the receiver must both be able to concentrate on the messages they send to each other without any distraction.

8. Improving communication

Some ways of improving communication are as follows:

- Listen without interrupting the sender.

- Show empathy at all times and try to understand.

- Try to stay focused on the conversation. Do not however, force the patient to continue if he/she becomes anxious or seems to wish to change the subject.

- Use the body language that indicates your interest and concern. Touch the patient if it seems appropriate. Lean forward, listen intently and maintain eye contact if it culturally acceptable.

- Offer factual information. This relieves anxiety. Do not offer your personal opinion. Assure the patient that you have professional discretion.

- Try to reflect the feelings and thoughts the patient is expressing by rephrasing questions and comments using their own words.

- Avoid unclear or misleading messages.

- Avoid giving long explanations.

- Give your co-workers your full attention when communicating with them.

- Ask questions to clarify unclear messages.

- Do not interrupt until the sender has completed the message.

- Provide a quiet environment without distractions.

- Be convincing wen communicating [17].

9. Communicating with patients

There are several points to be kept in mind when communicating with patients. The first point is that you are there to provide care and support to the patient.

- Be open, respectful and gracious in all your interactions with the patient and keep his/her cultural preferences in mind.

- Answer nurses' bells promptly.

- Make sure you have the patients' attention when communicating.

- Use words that are non-threatening – explain what you would like to do and do not give orders to the patient.

- Use simple, understandable phrases, not medical terms as most patients do not understand these terms.

- Speak clearly and courteously.

- Use a pleasant and normal tone of voice to the hard of hearing.

- Always stand so that the patient can see the nurse's face when communicating, as lip reading is part of all normal hearing.

- Use body language that is appropriate.

- Explain facts and procedures before donning a mask that covers the wearer's mouth and lower face.

- Be alert to the patient's needs. Allow time for answers to your requests and to answer patient's questions [17].

10. Communicating by phone

Nurses often communicate over the phone with patients, family members and colleagues and this can lead to misunderstandings. The way in which the pone is answered and a message is interpreted needs special skills because the body language of the person at the other end of the phone line cannot be seen. When answering the phone or making a call:

- Always speak clearly into the mouthpiece of the phone.

- Offer a greeting for example, good morning or good afternoon.

- Identify the unit or place of work.

- Identify yourself by indicating who you are and where you are phoning from.

- Identify the person to whom you are speaking.

- Politely listen to the message and make notes if you think you may not remember all the information.

- If you are asked to call another person, note the date, time, caller's name and telephone number together with the message.

- Date and sign the message [17].

11. Assertive communication

The skill of assertiveness is important to nurses. Nurses are expected to be the patients' advocates. So, they need to have the assertive communication skills in order to be able to be patients' advocates. Assertiveness enables a person to be honest with him/herself and in relationships with others. Assertiveness helps to enhance relationships, avoid power games and is a vehicle for clear outcomes. Hargis as cited by van Niekerk identifies four elements of assertive communication [8]:

- **Content** – where the rights of the people involved are embedded gently in the statement. This could be done by using an explanation, empathy for the listener, and praise for the listener, an apology for the consequence for the listener or a compromise that is favorable to both people.

- **Covert elements** – where the speaker is able to recognize their rights and the rights of the listener in the communication process. These include respect, expressing feelings, having your own priorities, being able to say 'no', being able to make mistakes and choosing to say nothing.

- **Process** – concerned with how people express themselves assertively. Is their body language, intonation and choice of language reflective of a confident assertive person? Are the processes that make up communication congruent, in keeping with what is being said? The process also involves managing the setting so that people are not embarrassed, or the noise levels are kept to a minimum. Increasing the likelihood of assertive communication happening again involves feedback to the listener to show that their accomplishment is appreciated.

- **Non-verbal cues** – gesture, touch, proxemics and posture – also need to reflect confidence, regard and respect for self and others.

12. Therapeutic interactions

Therapeutic interactions are purposeful as opposed to social. Social interaction entertains the participants, but in a professional situation, the nurse usually has a clinical objective that he/she wants to achieve with communication. The nurses therefore, decides on the purpose of the interaction before or shortly after it begins. The following purposes are common in nursing:

- **Assess a patient**: The nurse wants to know more about a patient to identify his/her problems. This type of conversation can be a structured interview using an interview schedule. The purpose of this conversation is always a better understanding of the patient.

- **Instruct a patient**: Patient instruction may vary from an informal conversation during which few facts are conveyed to an elaborate instruction session.

- **Problem solving**: If a patient discuss his/her problems with a nurse, the nurse helps the patient to analyze the problem, consider possible alternative ways of handling it and how to decide which way is the best. Problem solving is done with the patients and not for them.

- **Give emotional support**: The presence of an empathetic nurse, that is, one who can enter into the patient's shoes and understand the patient's experience, is immensely supportive of the patient. Emotional support alleviates the loneliness of the patient's experience of illness and increases his/her dignity [17].

13. Guidelines for successful therapeutic interactions

After the purpose of the therapeutic interaction has been established, the following guidelines assist in conducting a successful interaction:

13.1. Maintaining a low-authority profile

The nurse must strive to maintain a low-authority profile at the beginning of the conversation. As the conversation progresses, the nurse can use more directive techniques to find out specific information. There are usually differences in age, sex, occupation, cultural background, moral and religious convictions between the nurse and the patient. These differences make it impossible for the nurse to fully understand the patient's behavior and reactions. It is therefore, important for the nurse to understand and accept differences in patients' cultures and beliefs. When in doubt, check with the patient. If trust is established, patient will be willing to teach the nurse.

13.2. Use of understandable language

The nurse should determine the patient's level of understanding and if necessary change the use of language, comments and questions. Using the terminology which the patient does not understand can also frighten the patient and make him/her think that he/she has a more serious problem than he/she originally wanted help for. At the same time, the patient could give incorrect information because due to confusion, he/she may give affirmative answers to questions about symptoms that he/she has not actually experienced [18]. Nurses should share their aims with patients before expecting them to participate in the interaction. They should understand that there is a mutual understanding of each other's point of departure. In an assessment interview, the nurse can, for instance, say: "Mr Jones, I would like to give you information on how to lose weight so as to bring down you high blood pressure, but I first need to find out what you already know about the condition". It is not only important that the patients understand what nurses expect from the conversation; it is also essential that nurses understand the patients and convey this understanding before they participate in the conversation. When providing emotional support, this understanding is often all that is necessary. For nurses to understand patients, they must encourage them to talk – not just about facts, but also about their feelings. The nurse must listen more than speak, both to what the patient is saying verbally and what is being said non-verbally. Having listened carefully, the nurse then concentrates and responds empathetically to the patients' feelings. Only when the nurse has a reasonably complete understanding of the patient's situation and has communicated this understanding, can she proceed to interventions, such as giving information or solving a problem.

13.3. Tailor the message to the totality of the person

Saying something does not necessary mean that the message has been received and understood. It is the responsibility of the nurse to ensure that the person with whom he/she is conversing understands the message. To ensure this, the message has to be adapted to the language, culture and socio-economic status of the patient. The emotional or physical condition of patients may also make it difficult for them to receive long of complicated messages or even any message. There may also be other disturbances in the immediate environment for example, noise that can make the patient not to hear or understand the message. The message must also be adapted to the age of the patient [10].

13.4. Validate the interpretation with the patient

Validation means that you ask the patient whether your interpretation is correct or not. You therefore, ask him/her to confirm your understanding of what he/she said. Many misunderstandings arise because people interpret other people's words without checking their interpretation. The nurse should try to eliminate misunderstandings in the conversations by checking meaning with the patient.

13.5. Active listening

Active listening means concentrating all your senses and thoughts on the speaker. One can usually deduce whether a person is listening actively by looking at the following non-verbal indicators:

- Is the eye contact maintained with the person who is speaking?

- Are the body and face turned towards the speaker?

It is, of course, also clear from the verbal responses:

- Are there regular verbal responses, even if these consist only of encouraging sounds?

- Does the response indicate understanding, not only of the facts, but also of the feelings and the implications of the facts?

It is much easier to speak than to listen. Nurses are, in general, very active people, who want help b acting quickly. To 'just listen' without expressing opinions or offering advice is therefore, often not in their nature. Active listening is a valuable skill to acquire [10, 17, 18].

13.6. Evaluate own communication

In the interest of nurse–patient relationship, it is essential that they ascertain whether their communication has been successful. The following criteria can be used:

- **Simplicity**: Say what you want to say concisely and without using difficult or unfamiliar terms.

- **Clarity**: Say precisely what you want to say without digressing, and support your verbal message with non-verbal indicators.

- **Relevance**: Make sure that your message suits the situation, the time and the person you are speaking to.

- **Adaptability**: Adapt your response to the clues the patient that the patient gives you.

- **Respect**: Always show respect for the individuality and dignity of the person you are speaking to [17].

14. Therapeutic communication techniques

Table 1 gives an overview of therapeutic communication techniques and provides examples of each technique [10, 13].

General area of issue	Therapeutic communication techniques	Rationale	Examples
To obtain information	Make broad opening remarks	This gives the patient the freedom to choose what he/she wishes to talk about	"Please tell me more about yourself"
	Use open-ended questions	This type of question allows the patient to talk about his/her views about the subject. In this way, what the patient sees as important, what his/her intellectual capacity is and how well-orientated he/she is, becomes clear. This encourages the patient to say more and does not limit answers to a 'yes' or 'no'	"How did you experience the pain?" "You say you felt dizzy, and then…" "Tell me more about that"
	Share observations and thoughts	This shows that you are aware of what is happening to the patient and encourages him/her to talk about it	"You seem to be upset"
	Confrontation	This entails confronting the patient with an observation you have made and assess his/her reaction to it. This technique is useful when verbal and non-verbal communication do not match	"You say that your ankle is very painful, but you do not react when I bend the ankle. How is it possible?"
	Reflection	This means that you repeat what the patient said in the same or different words. This shows you are involved in what the patient is saying and that he/she should talk more about a specific point, or explain further	Patient: "It is sore". Nurse: "Very painful?"
	Encourage description	This is used to obtain more information about patient's views and feelings	"Tell me how it happened"
	Validate what is being said	This is to make sure that you understand the patient correctly	"Do I understand you correctly when you say…"
	Offer your presence	The nurse offers his/her attention and interest without making demands	"I will be with you until they come to fetch you for the operation in theater"
	Summarizing	By organizing and checking what the patient has said, especially after a detailed discussion. This technique is used to indicate that a specific part of the discussion is coming to an end and that if the patient wishes to say any more, she should do so	"You went for a walk and then you felt the sharp chest pains, which radiated down your arm"
	Use of interpretation	Draw a conclusion from the information you have gathered and discuss it with your patient to see whether it is true. The patient can then disagree with it, or confirm that your conclusions are true	"You must have been exhausted after walking a long distance from home to the hospital"

General area of issue	Therapeutic communication techniques	Rationale	Examples
To give support	Supportive remarks	Make supportive remarks to encourage the patient to participate in the conversation. Show that you are listening	"Yes…." "Mmmm…" "Go on, I am listening"
	Appropriately touch the patient	Touch can assure the patient that the nurse cares and is present	Hold his/her hand. Consider the cultural belief and comfort of the patient before touching
	Paraphrasing	This conveys understanding of the patient's basic message	"It sounds as though the most important problem is the diet"
To assist in analysis and problem solving	Acknowledge the person	This promotes a sense of dignity	"Good morning Mr. Jones"
	Sequencing	This helps the patient to see the connection between the parts of an occurrence. To effectively assess the patient's needs, the nurse often needs to know the time frame within which symptom sand /or problems developed or occurred	"Did you experience this sharp pain before or after eating?"
	Ask for clarification	This helps the nurse to understand and the patient to communicate more clearly	"What do you mean by everybody?"
	Ask for alternatives	This stimulates creative thought and promotes finding solutions	"What else can you try?"
	Use of transition	This is used to guide the conversation to another subject, without losing the continuity of the conversation	"It seems to me that you have solved the problem of poor appetite, but I would like to hear more about your diabetes. How long have you been aware of this illness?"
	Comparison	Use of examples and comparisons to concrete objects. In this way, a vague or abstract concept can be more easily explained	"Does the pain feel like a sharp or a blunt object that hits you?"
	Use silence	This gives the patient the chance to think, and/or to his/her organize thoughts. Silence also give a nurse an opportunity to observe the patient. However, the nurse should avoid silences that last too long because they can make the patient anxious	
To instruct the patient	Give information	This explains information and puts it at the patient's disposal	"After the operation, you will have a drainage tube"
	Orientate the patient towards reality	When the patient interprets something incorrectly, the nurse draws his/her attention to reality	"I am not your daughter, I am Nurse Jones"
	Query what the patient says	The patient's observation is called into question without belittling him/her, or arguing about it	Are you sure about that?"
	Withhold social reward	Do not give social approval to wrong behavior so as not to encourage a repeat of the wrong behavior	Do not smile, nod or agree when the patient jeopardizes his/her recovery with wrong behavior
	Give social reward	Reward behavior that promotes health to encourage a repeat of the correct behavior	Nod is approval at a patient with a weight problem who declines to eat a heavy meal

Table 1. Therapeutic communication techniques.

15. Counter-productive communication techniques

There are certain counter-productive communication techniques that the nurse should avoid as they do not assist in the recovery of the patient and do not have any therapeutic value. **Table 2** shows counter-productive communication techniques, explains why these should be avoided and gives examples [10, 18].

Non-therapeutic techniques	Rationale	Examples
Inappropriate reassurance	The nurse attempts to brush aside the patient's aside the patient's worry by acting as though it is unnecessary or inappropriate. Reassurance is not based on fact or real certainty. This helps the nurse more than it helps the patient	"Do not worry; everything will be fine"
Passing judgment	The nurse passes judgment on the patient's behavior, thoughts or feelings and in doing so, places herself in the position of an adversary or a person who knows better and more	"As a Christian, I do not think you should terminate this pregnancy"
Giving advice	The nurse tells the patient how he/she ought to feel, think or act. This implies that she has the correct information and knows better than the patient. This is particularly problematic when the advice is based on limited assessment and knowledge of the patient and the situation	"I think you must..."
Closed questions	These questions require only a single word as an answer when specific information is needed. If this type of question is used often, the patient are less inclined to give the information and may be interpreted as an interrogation	"Do you feel any pain in your arm?"
'Why' questions	These questions demand that the patient explains behavior, feelings or thoughts that he/she often does not understand himself or herself. These questions are often asked early in a conversation when the nurse cannot even be certain that the patient wants to explain himself of herself to the nurse	"Why are you upset?"
Offering platitudes	This is stereotyped expression of something the patient is in any case aware of and which, therefore, helps little. This is similar to giving advice	"Everybody goes through this in life"
Defensiveness	The nurse tries to defend someone or something the patient criticized. This places the nurse and the patient on opposite sides and does not promote further openness on the part of the patient	"We are very short-staffed; so we cannot help everyone at the same time"

Table 2. Non-therapeutic communication techniques that should be avoided.

16. Conclusion

Promoting effective communication in health care is demanding and challenging because of the nature of the work environment. Nurses who have received training in communication skills communicate effectively and show increased confidence in communicating with patients. Many nurses choose to work in other countries, providing an opportunity to broaden their experience and knowledge. However, it is important that nurses who have the opportunity to work in other countries develop communication skills, cultural awareness and sensitivity before arriving. For example, in China talking about death is taboo [19]. In South Africa, maintaining eye during communication may be regarded as being disrespectful by Black people [11]. This article provides a reflective account of the experiences of one of the authors of working overseas. This chapter provides the effective communication and interpersonal skills that enhance professional nursing practice and nursing relationships by explaining principles of communication, communication process, purpose of communication, types of communication, barriers to effective communication, models of communication and strategies of improving communication and guidelines for successful therapeutic interactions.

Acknowledgements

The author wishes to acknowledge the Durban University of Technology for funding this book chapter.

Conflict of interest

The author declares that there is no conflict of interest in this chapter.

Author details

Maureen Nokuthula Sibiya

Address all correspondence to: nokuthulas@dut.ac.za

Durban University of Technology, Durban, South Africa

References

[1] World Health Organization (WHO). Global strategic directions for strengthening nursing and midwifery 2016-2020. 2016. Geneva: WHO

[2] Mokoka KE, Ehlers VJ, Oosthuizen MJ. Factors influencing the retention of registered nurses in the Gauteng Province of South Africa. Curationis. 2011;34(1):1-9

[3] Mokoka E, Oosthuizen MJ, Ehlers VJ. Retaining professional nurses in South Africa: Nurse managers' perspectives. Health SA Gesondheid. 2010;15(1):1-9

[4] Neese B. Effective Communication in Nursing: Theory and Best Practices. [Internet]. 2015. Available from: http://online.seu.edu/effective-communication-in-nursing/ [Accessed: December 28, 2017]

[5] Bush H. Communication Skills for Nurses. [Internet]. 2016. Available from: https://www.ausmed.com/articles/communication-skills-for-nurses/ [Accessed: December 28, 2017]

[6] O'Hagan S, Manias E, Elder C, Pill J, Woodward-Kron R, McNamara T, Webb G, McColl G. What counts as effective communication in nursing? Evidence from nurse educators' and clinicians' feedback on nurse interactions with simulated patients. Journal of Advanced Nursing. 2013:1344-1355

[7] Sibiya MN. People management. In: Booyens S, Jooste K, Sibiya N, editors. Introduction to Health Services Management for the Unit Manager. 4th ed. Claremont: Juta and Company (Pty) Ltd; 2015. pp. 194-205. ISBN: 978-0-70218-866-4

[8] van Niekerk V. Relationship, helping and communication skills. In: van Rooyen, D, Jordan PJ, editors. Foundations of Nursing Practice: Fundamentals of Holistic Care. African Edition. 2nd ed. Edinburgh: Mosby Elsevier; 2016. pp. 181-207. ISBN: 978-0-7020-6628-3

[9] Jooste K. Effective leadership communication. In: Jooste K, editor. Leadership in Health Services Management. 2nd ed. Claremont: Juta and Company (Pty) Ltd; 2011. pp. 205-220. ISBN: 9-780702-180347

[10] Uys L. Interpersonal needs. In: Uys L, editor. Integrated Fundamental Nursing. 2nd ed. Cape Town: Pearson; 2017. pp. 453-571. ISBN: 978-1-775-95450-7

[11] du Plessis E, Jordaan EJ, Jali MN. Communication in a health care unit. In: Jooste K, editor. The Principles and Practice of Nursing and Health Care. Pretoria: Van Schaik Publishers; 2010. pp. 205-220. ISBN: 9-780627-027857

[12] Kai J, Beavan J, Faull C. Challenges of mediated communication, disclosure and patient autonomy in cross-cultural cancer care. British Journal of Cancer. 2011;105(7):918-924

[13] McCarthy J, Cassidy I, Margaret MG, Tuohy D. Conversations through barriers of language and interpretation. Bristish Journal of Nursing. 2013;22(6):335-340

[14] Tay LH, Ang E, Hegney D. Nurses' perceptions of the barriers in effective communication with inpatient cancer adults in Singapore. Journal of Clinical Nursing. 2012; 21(17-18):2647-2658

[15] Aslakson RA, Wyskiel R, Thornton I, Copley C, Shaffer D, Zyra M, Pronovost PJ. Nurse-perceived barriers to effective communication regarding prognosis and optimal end-of-life care for surgical ICU patients: A qualitative exploration. Journal of Palliative Medicine. 2012;15(8):910-915

[16] Helft PR, Chamness A, Terry C, Uhrich M. Oncology nurses' attitudes toward prognosis-related communication: A pilot mailed survey of oncology nursing society members. Oncology Nursing Forum. 2011;38(4):468-474

[17] Booyens L, Erasmus I, van Zyl M. The Auxiliary Nurse. 3rd ed. Cape Town: Juta and Company Ltd; 2013. 504 p. ISBN: 978-0-702 19-794-9

[18] Viljoen MJ, Sibiya N. History Taking and Physical Examination. 2nd ed. Cape Town: Pearson Education South Africa (Pty) Ltd; 2009. ISBN: 978-1-86891-976-5

[19] Zheng RS, Guo QH, Dong FQ, Owens RG. Chinese oncology nurses' experience on caring for dying patients who are in their final days: A qualitative study. International Journal of Nursing Studies. 2015;52(1):288-296

Nursing and Culture

Chapter 4

Transcultural Nursing

Vasfiye Bayram Değer

Additional information is available at the end of the chapter

http://dx.doi.org/10.5772/intechopen.74990

Abstract

Culture is defined as the sum of all the material and spiritual values created in the process of social development and the tools that are used to create and hand these values down to next generations and show the extent of the man's authority and control over their natural and social environment. The term "culture", which diversifies in each community and so is experienced differently, also affects the way individuals perceive the phenomena such as health, illness, happiness, sadness and the manner these emotions are experienced. The term health, whose nature and meaning is highly variable across different cultures requires care involving cultural recognition, valueing and practice. The nursing profession, which plays an important role in the health team, is often based on a cultural phenomenon. The cultural values, beliefs and practices of the patient are an integral part of holistic nursing care. The aim of nursing is to provide a wholly caring and humanistic service respecting people's cultural values and lifestyles. Nurses should offer an acceptable and affordable care for the individuals under the conditions of the day. Knowing what cultural practices are done in the target communities and identifying the cultural barriers to offering quality health care positively affects the caring process. Nurses should explore new ways of providing cultural care in multicultural societies, understand how culture affects health-illness definitions and build a bridge for the gap between the caring process and the individuals in different cultures.

Keywords: culture, health, nurse, transcultural nursing, health services

1. Introduction

It is useful to define the culture before discussing the term. According to the definition made by Turkish Language Institution Culture, the culture is described as the sum of all the material and spiritual values created in the process of social development and the tools that are used to create and hand these values down to next generations and show the extent of the man's authority and control over their natural and social environment [1].

According to another definition, the culture is the general total of beliefs, attitudes and behaviors, customs and traditions, learned and shared values, and sustains its existence through learning and teaching of attitudes, actions and role models [2].

As it can be understood from these definitions, culture is a non-written link from the past to the present day, bridging the individuals in society. As a phenomenon, The term "culture," which diversifies in each community and so is experienced differently, also affects the way individuals perceive the phenomena such as health, illness, happiness, sadness and the manner these emotions are experienced [3].

Culture is a relative concept that varies according to health cultures as well as affecting the perception of health [4].

Health is determined by biological and environmental factors as well as by cultural practices [5].

Culture affects many aspects of human life, such as parental attitudes, child rearing patterns, how to speak, what language to speak, how to dress, believe, treat patients, what to do with and how to feed them and to deal with funerals [6, 7].

Individuals' health behaviors and health perceptions are regarded inseparable from each other. Communities having endeavored to maintain their cultural characteristics for centuries have passed down this on their health behaviors and strived for finding cures to their health problems in their cultural lives. Types of food, cooking methods, sleeping habits, dressing patterns, forms of treatment of diseases, housing and residence, perception of diseases, modes of acceptance of innovations are characteristics varying from culture to culture and intertwined with culture. It is known that people cannot act independently of the culture they live in [8].

Culture is influential at many levels in health, ranging from the formation of new diagnostic groups, to the diagnosis of disease to the determination of what is called a disease or not symptoms and disease cues [6, 7].

However, in almost all regions of the world, wars, ethnic conflicts, repressive regimes, environmental and economic crises along with globalization have forced many people to abandon their country and migrate in their country or to immigrate other countries as refugees. As a result, multicultural populations comprised of individuals, families and groups from different cultures and subcultures are rapidly emerging all around the world [9–11].

2. Cultural factors affecting health and disease

In order to improve the health behaviors of the community, cultural factors affecting health behavior and health care services need to be clearly recognized [12, 13].

The individuals' beliefs about health, attitudes and behaviors, past experiences, treatment practices, in short their culture, play a vital role in improving health, preventing and treating diseases [14].

Cultural variables can be motivational factors in health-disease relationships, [8].

2.1. Cultural factors/variables can be listed as in the following list

1. Socioeconomic status

2. Family pattern

3. Gender roles and responsibilities

4. Marriage patterns

5. Sexual behavior

6. Preventive patterns

7. Population policy

8. Pregnancy and birth practices

9. Body

10. Nutrition

11. Dressing/wearing

12. Personal hygiene

13. Housing arrangements

14. General health regulations

15. Professions

16. Religion

17. Habits

18. Culture-induced stress

19. Status of immigrants

20. Substance use

21. Leisure time habits of

22. Pets and birds

23. Self-healing strategies and therapies [8].

3. Health culture

Today, health-related cultural traits are under the influence of a medical approach that may be considered as highly conservative almost all around the world. There is an increasing tendency to perceive and evaluate health and disease-related processes explained in medical terms. The rigid medical approach, engaged in extending human life with costly inventions, with a narrow level of knowledge and practices, makes it impossible for individuals to use the potential for qualified living. Modern medicine overwhelms the will of people to experience their own facts and solve their problems. On the other hand, the concept of health should be regarded as a dynamic phenomenon in life and be removed from some patterns of thought. Hence, healthcare should be assessed with a comprehensive understanding of culture in order to promote the art of living healthily among people [15].

Individuals who embrace contemporary public health, evaluate health with a holistic approach, give the other individuals an opportunity to participate in their health care issues, and have the potential to solve problems with appropriate preferences can only be the output of cultural constructs supporting health, values, knowledge, attitudes, behaviors and norms. Health culture is concerned with every individual's or the society's patterns of living, celebrating, being happy in life, suffering and dying. It is not enough for the individual to acquire only health-related information, but basic skills such as comprehending health-related values, developing a healthy lifestyle and self-evaluation must be developed. The main purpose of developing health culture is to raise the level of health in the country scale. This can only be ensured by the fact that health education standards be established by well-trained and conscious individuals into practice with the help of their knowledge and skills [15].

4. Transcultural healthcare

It is vital that health services are also appropriate for the target cultures to the extent that they are compatible with contemporary medical understanding. People's beliefs and practices are part of the culture of the society in which they live. Cultural characteristics should be seen as a dynamic factor of health and disease. In order to be able to provide better health care, it is necessary to at least understand how the group receiving care perceives and responds to disease and health, and what cultural factors lie behind their behaviors [7, 13, 16–20].

Unless health care initiatives are based on cultural values, it will be impossible to achieve the goal and the care provided will be incomplete and fail [2, 21].

For this reason, healthcare providers should try to understand the cultural structure of a society. Health workers must collect cultural data to understand the attitudes of towards coping with illness, health promotion and protection [2, 21].

Cultural differences and health beliefs have been recognized for many years as prior knowledge in practice. Despite that, cultural health care is unfortunately not part of a routine or common health practice. Knowing cultural beliefs related to health can enable us to build a framework for data collection in health care [2, 22].

Today, health policies focus primarily on the prevention of health-related inequalities and discrimination, especially ethnic characteristics. In order for the societies to regulate health care that will meet the needs of different groups in terms of culture, all health team members must be equipped with the necessary knowledge and skills [23, 24].

5. Understanding transcultural nursing

The term health, with its changing nature and meanings from one culture to another, requires care, including cultural recognition, value and practice. The main element in the transcultural approach in which every health professional has an active role is the individual. The transcultural approach can be applied at all levels of health care institutions; but nurses are in a privileged position in this approach. According to Leininger's model, only nurses can provide transcultural health services. Because the main aim of nursing is to provide a caring service that respects people's cultural values and lifestyles. Nurses should offer acceptable, affordable and culturally suitable care to individuals under the conditions of the day [2].

Knowing what cultural practices are applied in the societies receiving healthcare services and identifying the cultural barriers to accessing health care services positively affects the caring process [25].

The nursing profession, which plays an important role in the health team, is a cultural phenomenon. The patient's cultural values, beliefs and practices are an integral part of holistic nursing care [26, 27].

The nurses should explore new ways of providing cultural care in multicultural societies, understand how cultures affect health-disease definitions, and bridge the gap between care for individuals in different cultures [13, 28, 29].

Transcultural nursing provides effective nursing care to meet the cultural needs of individuals, families and groups [30].

The concept of "Transcultural Nursing" derived from the need to care for individuals in different cultures in nursing was first used by Madeleine Leininger in 1979 [30–32].

In addition to Leininger, a pioneer model of transcultural nursing, many nurses worked in the field of cultural care. Giger and Davidhazar developed the "Cross-Cultural Diagnosis Model" to assess various variables related to health and illness and provide a practical diagnostic tool for nursing so that culturally competent care could be offered [33].

Campinha-Bacote described the cultural competence model [34].

Culturally competent nurses are in contact with cultural experiences and aware of their own personality traits and contribute to socio-cultural knowledge in nursing care by providing individualized care [35].

Nurses who are aware of cultural differences and the effects of these differences on the health of the individual enhance the therapeutic environment by communicating more effectively with the patients [13].

The role and significance of transcultural nursing has been increasingly recognized in the world challenged by cultural diversity. Cultural differences can be seen among ethnic groups as well as within any ethnic group [36].

It has been reported that cultural differences may exist among individuals who live in the same or different regions in Turkey [37].

Although studies on cross-cultural nursing care in our country are limited, several studies have examined the views of nursing and midwifery students regarding patient care [37–39].

In a study conducted, the views of nurses working in two different hospitals on the cultural problems they faced in patient care were compared [11, 36].

In recent years, it has been recognized that nurses must explore new ways of providing cultural care in culturally diverse societies, understand how culture affects disease-health definitions, and act as a bridge between the biomedical system and care for individuals in different cultures [2, 40].

The nature and importance of providing culturally sensitive nursing services is multidimensional, including individual and professional aspects. The transcultural approach allows nurses to broaden their horizons and perspectives in addition to making them competent in offering creative care to individuals. Culturally based approaches and knowledge can enhance both the nurse's and the patient's self-esteem [2, 41, 42].

The American Nurses Association (ANA) refers to three reciprocal interactions: the culture of the individual (patient), the culture of the nurse, and the culture of the environment in relation to the patient-nurse:

Culture of the individual: When nurses understand the specific factors affecting individual health behaviors, they will be more successful in meeting their needs [2].

Individuals' beliefs about health, culture, past illness/health experiences form a wholistic structure and play a vital role in improving the health of individuals [43].

Culture is influential in how people think, speak the language, how to dress, believe, treat their patients and how to feed them and what to do with their funerals etc. Moreover, it plays a significant role in a variety of aspects such as new diagnostic methods, prognosis, symptomatic patterns and determination of whether there is an illness or not [7].

Culture of the nurse: The only factor influencing the patient-nurse relationship is not the patient himself/herself. The nurses' own customs and traditions, beliefs and values are also important in transcultural relationships. The nurse's self-awareness can be the starting point to understand the patient culturally.

Culture of the environment: The last element of the transcultural trio is the culture of the environment. The environment is an integral part of the culture. Individuals as physical, ecological, sociopolitical and cultural beings are continuously interacting with each other. Nurses may have to intervene in the patient and family relationship because of frequent bureaucratic arrangements and procedures. The transcultural approach should be considered in a wide range of subjects, starting from asking if there are any religious practices to be followed or done by the patient during the hospitalization, and writing the signs in the hospital in two different languages [13].

6. The significance of cultural competence

It is essential for nurses to be able to offer appropriate holistic care to patients from different cultures and to know how the transcultural approach is to be put into practice, as it provides guidance on how to behave in the case of these situations.

Transcultural nursing is sensitive to the needs of families, groups and individuals who are representatives of groups with different cultures in a community or society. This sensitive approach provides support for the individual in achieving the well-being and happiness [2].

Culturally sensitive nursing practices involve the identification of cultural needs, the understanding of cultural links between family and individuals to provide care without affecting the cultural belief system of the family, and the use of emotional strategies for caregivers and patients to reach reciprocal goals. Building therapeutic relationships, offering appropriate and responsive care and treatment can be accomplished through transcultural nursing approach [2].

It is necessary for nurses to recognize individuals in their own cultural patterns, examine them in their own culture, and take these into account in the nursing approach [2, 7, 22].

Nursing is a developing profession that can continuously adapt to changing situations. Changes in social rules and expectations, the advent of new medical treatments, and improvements in technical systems have helped shape contemporary nursing practices [4, 44, 45].

Nursing has been significantly influenced by the fact that an increasing number of societies around the world have become multicultural and cultural specific care has been recognized [4].

The concept of cultural competence is a relatively new concept commonly used in the academic disciplines from the beginning of 1989 [4, 46, 47].

In multicultural societies, health care professionals need to be culturally competent, which is expected by the society. Interest in cultural competence has been manifested in the studies conducted on the cultural characteristics of the patients [46].

The nurses' understanding of the cultures of patient groups is very important for the provision of meaningful effective nursing care [48].

The study performed by Chenowethm et al. titled as the "Cultural Proficiency and Nursing Care: With an Australian Perspective" and Giger and Davidhizar's study titled as "Culturally

Adequate Care: The Afghan, Afghan Origin American and the Importance of Understanding Islamic Cultural and Islamic Religion" can be cited as examples of conducted research on this subject [4, 33, 49].

Providing culturally adequate care is an obligation imposed by increased cultural diversity and disclosure of identities, an understanding of home care and inequalities in health care. Cultural competence is a dynamic, variable and continuous process. Although cultural competence is a basic component of nursing practice, this concept has not been clearly explained or analyzed but defined in many ways. At times, various terms such as "transcultural nursing", "culturally appropriate nursing care" or "culturally sensitive nursing care" were used instead of the term cultural competence [46].

The literature review reveals that there is a common definition of cultural competence the term among researchers and a general consensus on the term. For example, the concepts of "ethnic nursing care", "cultural care", "cultural appropriateness" or "culturally appropriate care" are seen as terms close to cultural adequacy [4, 47].

Cultural competence is the application of knowledge, skills, attitudes, and personal manners anticipated from nurses to provide services and care appropriate to the cultural characteristics of the patients.

Başalan İz ve Bayık Temel reported that Vydelingum [47] made use of Murphy and Macleod-Clark, Bond, Kadron-Edgren and Jones, Spence, Blackford's findings in his study. In Murphy and Macleod-Clark's study on ethnocentric views, it was stated by nurses that patients from a minority group were generally regarded as a problem and these patients were perceived as inappropriate for daily routine, and there was lack of holistic care among nurses working to develop a therapeutic relationship with minority groups. Bond, Kadron-Edgren and Jones conducted a study evaluating the knowledge and attitudes of nursing students and professional nurses regarding patients from different cultures. This study has shown that undergraduate and post-graduate nursing programs are partially limited in terms of the knowledge and skills about special cultural groups. Spence, in his study on nurses' experiences in caring for people from other cultures in New Zealand found that they experienced tension and anxiety when they encountered with an odd case. The subject of cultural well-being and nursing approaches in nursing education was reported in a study carried out by Blackford in Australia. The necessity of care structured under the roof of the white race culture has revealed that it does not consider the health care culture. The lack of cultural adequacy in the care of patients from different cultures has been recognized as an great challenge to all these studies. Cultural conflict has been shown as an output of ethnocentric focus, resulting in a lack of cultural competence, misunderstanding, lack of confidence, communication and obstacles to establishing a positive relationship [4].

The nurse experiencing cultural conflict must first recognize his/her subconscious cultural behaviors in order to understand the reason for the cultural conflict [13].

In a cultural conflict, the nurse can respond negatively from the cultural perspective in the following ways:

- **Ethnocentrism:** It refers the individual's interpretation of other cultures in terms of their own culture based on their own cultural heritage.

- **Stereotyping:** The acceptance of the same characteristics of individuals or group members without considering individual differences.

- **Cultural blindness:** A symptom of not paying attention to expressing cultural diversity.

- **Cultural imposition:** The situation emerges at a time when the nurse expects the patient to comply with his/her cultural norms or the norms of the health institution. The nurse may think, "You have to follow my hospital's rule and comply with our procedures here."

- **Cultural conflict:** When a nurse, patient and family have different values, exhibit different behaviors, conflicts may arise in the case of differences in beliefs and traditions. However, the expected professional attitude from the nurse is cultural relativism. Cultural relativism means recognizing and understanding the individual's culture in its own structure, without referring to other norms and judgments. The nurse approaching the patient with cultural relativism has a clear view of the characteristics of cultures, diversity of beliefs and practices in different environments resulting from different social needs [2].

6.1. In culturally sensitive care, there are three major approaches reducing cultural conflicts to minimum. These are listed below

1. The individual/patient's own perspective and cultural beliefs must be respected and recognized.

2. The nurse should be competent and authorized to carry out professional actions and make decisions.

3. The nurse should help the individual to develop new patterns to lead a satisfying and healthy life in the case of harmful behaviors [50].

The nursing care plan must be individual, holistic and contemporary. Interpreters or religious leaders may need to be included in the caring plan if there are any linguistic problems. The patient's view on the cause of his or her illness is also a key element in planning the care [49].

In preparing the nursing care plan, basic principles related to culturally sensitive nursing practices can be followed.

6.2. Basic principles related to culturally sensitive nursing practices are described below

- The importance and influence of the culture should be considered,

- Cultural differences should be valued and respected,

- Cultural influences in the manners of individuals should be understood,

- An empathic approach should be put into action towards individuals with cultural diversity,

- Individuals' cultures should be respected,

- Health professionals should be patient with individuals in cultural issues,

- Individuals' behaviors should be thoroughly analyzed,

- Cultural knowledge should be increased and enhanced,

- Adaptation and orientation programs about cultural diversity should be offered [2, 7, 22].

6.3. The scope of cultural nursing practice

The scope of cultural nursing practice can be:

- identification of cultural needs

- understanding the cultural connections of the individual and the

- using emotional strategies for the caregivers and the patients to reach the reciprocal goals

Thus, the cultural approach will guide the nurses in planning nursing interventions. In this case, nursing care can be provided without harming the cultural belief system of the family [13, 51].

This short review provides the basis for a deeper cultural assessment that the nurse can do in the future. The nurse has the opportunity to communicate effectively with the individual through brief cultural assessment data collected [7, 13, 22, 52].

Nurses should make cultural evaluations when they first communicate with individuals. This evaluation may be in-depth, or a brief review that will form the basis for an in-depth assessment to be done later. In a brief review, several questions about health practices, diet, religious preference, ethnic background and family can be asked to the individual. This short review provides the basis for a deeper cultural assessment to be done by the nurse in the future. Thus, the nurse has a chance to communicate effectively with the individual through brief cultural data [7, 13, 22, 52].

6.4. Data collection

1. Demographic data

   - Regional population density

   - Population density entering the region

   - Age distribution of the residents in the region

- Distribution of demographics such as education, job, income etc.
- The national origin of the population living in the region

2. Traditional health beliefs

- Definition of illness
- Definition of health
- Health-related behaviors
- Reasons for your illness
- Poor eating habits/nutrition
- Bad eating arrangements
- Viruses, bacteria and other organisms
- A punishment/curse from Allah (the God)
- Being affected by the evil eyes
- Magic, charm, spell or jealousy
- Witchcraft
- Environmental changes
- Sorrow or loss
- Excessive or little labor

3. Methods for maintaining health

4. Health protection methods

5. Methods of restoring health-home treatments/household recipes

6. Utilization of health care resources and visitations

7. Traditional healers favored by sick people

8. Health beliefs and practices related to childbirth

9. Health beliefs and practices related to raising children

10. Traditional practices and ceremonies arranged for dying individuals and related to death

In addition to recognizing the cultural characteristics of the community, by depending on these data, nurses should recognize traditional medicines, places of worship and sacredness, and other such organizations and, if possible, should visit and observe such places in order to identify the service group.

6.5. The issues to be considered which enable nurses to make cultural assessment include the following

1. The nurses should be knowledgeable about the community receiving care services provided by themselves.

2. The nurses should identify the social gathering environments such as schools, hospitals, places of worship of the community they serve care.

3. The nurses should define the specific areas they want to focus on prior to cultural evaluation.

4. The nurses should determine the strategies that can help them collect data about cultural values.

5. The nurses should define the items that may act as bridges between the cultures.

6. The nurses should be able to ask appropriate questions without hurting the individuals.

7. The nurses should cooperate with colleagues and other health workers.

8. The nurses should discuss with the community leaders, whether official or non-official, about cultural characteristics deemed important in the lifestyle of the society.

9. The nurses should not resort to unethical traps to make an early generalization based on the cultural data of the society.

10. The nurses should be honest, open and sincere towards the individuals and the self.

11. The nurses should obtain both objective and subjective data and verify them to be correct before implementing nursing care [7, 13].

Additionally, the nurses should at least learn some relevant vocabulary and common phrases used in caregiving that will facilitate communication [7, 13].

6.6. Transcultural nursing focuses on four major concepts below

1. Nurses are transcultural care personnel.

2. An individual is considered as a cultural asset and cannot be separated from his/her own cultural heritage and background.

3. Environment is a structure or framework

4. Transcultural care is a sensitive nursing care service addressing to the needs of individuals from different cultural groups [18].

A manual of guidelines has been prepared by International Nurses Association (ICN), American Nursing Academy, Transcultural Nursing Association, with the aim of creating a common language for nursing practice all over the world and providing a holistic and cultural content care that respects social equality, justice and individual differences. There are 12 items in the manual given in the following:

1. Social Justice and Equality

2. Critical Perspective

3. Cultural Awareness

4. Cultural Based Care

5. Cultural Based Health Care Systems and Organizations

6. Patient Advocacy and Empowerment

7. Multicultural Workforce

8. Cultural Based Care in Education and Training

9. Intercultural Communication

10. Intercultural Leadership

11. Policy Development

12. Evidence Based Practices and Research [3, 53].

7. The history of transcultural nursing

The foundations of transcultural nursing were laid in the mid-1950s. In nursing, Peplau first mentioned in 1950 that the cultures were an important variable affecting mental health. The growing interest in Leininger's transcultural nursing model has begun with population changes and migration. Leininger tried to promote transcultural nursing movements. Much more attention was paid to the care of individuals from different cultures in the 1960s. Since 1960s, nurses have been carrying out studies aimed at providing particularly cultural care to people from all communities/cultures. In 1962, King stated that psychopathological behaviors differ from culture to culture. In 1969, the International Council of Nursing (ICN) began using cultural content in nursing. The Transcultural Nursing Society (TCNS) was established in 1974 to train nurses in this area.

This organization aims to provide the nurses and other health care professionals with the basic knowledge necessary to develop cultural skills in culturally sensitive practice, education, research and management [2].

Since 1989, "Journal of Transcultural Nursing" has been published, aiming to train nurses about transcultural care and improve their practice. Evidence-based studies have been conducted in this area. Today, there are about 25 books and over 800 articles covering research, theory and applications related to transcultural nursing [2].

This is a promising field of study with which Turkish nurses have recently started to be familiar. Now that globalization is inevitable, studies on transcultural care practices will broaden the horizons of Turkish nurses and the others all around the world.

In addition to Leininger, a pioneer model of transcultural nursing, many nurses worked in the field of cultural care including Boyle, Campinha-Bacote, Yahle Langenkamp, Giger and Davidhizar, Juntunen, Leuning, Swiggum et al., Purnell, Ryan, Carlton and Ali.

Among these, there are researchers arguing that the models and theories of two modelists (Giger and Davidhizar and Purnell) who do myriads of studies on cultural care are extremely simple, comprehensible and suitable for use in many different fields and cultures [5].

8. Transcultural nursing care models

8.1. Cultural competence models

1. Burchum JLR; Cultural competence: Evolutionary dimension.

2. Campinha-Bacote J; Cultural competence in providing health care services: Culturally adequate care model.

3. Cross T., Bazron B; Dennis K., Isaacs M.; Towards a culturally adequate care process: Effective services for minority children with emotionally serious illness.

4. Kim-Godwin YS; Clarke PN & Barton L.; Providing culturally adequate public care model.

5. Leininger MM; The differences in cultural care and the theory of universality.

6. Leininger M; Cultural care theory and ethnocentric research method.

7. Leininger M; Evaluation of culture care for appropriate and adequate practices.

8. Orque M.; Orque's ethnic/cultural system: Conceptual framework for ethnic nursing care.

9. Pacquiao DF; Cultural competence in ethical decision making.

10. Papadopoulos I. & Lees S; Training culturally competent researchers.

11. Purnell LD. & Amp; Paulanka BJ; Ppur model for cultural competence.

12. Suh EE; Cultural competence model through evolutionary concept analysis.

13. Wells M; Beyond cultural competence: a model for individual and institutional cultural development [4, 46].

8.2. Cultural assessment models

1. Giger JN. & Davidhizar RE; Transcultural nursing; Evaluation and intervention

2. Spector RE; Cultural difference in health and disease.

8.3. Cultural assessment guidelines

1. Andrews MM; Culturally adequate nursing care.

2. Andrews MM; History of health and cultural competence in physical examination.

3. Bloch B; Bloch's assessment guide for ethnic/cultural diversity.

4. Boyle JS & Andrews MM; Andrews/Boyle assessment guide.

5. Spector RE; Cultural care: guidelines for inheritance, assessment and health traditions [4, 46].

The conceptualization of the cultural competence model in nursing has emerged after 1989. Leininger, Campinha-Bacote, Giger and Davidhizar, Orque, Purnell and Paulanka, Spector, Andrews and Boyle are regarded as the pioneers contributing to the accumulation of the relevant data. Orque is a leading figure in developing a cultural model for nursing with "the conceptual framework of the ethnic system". The use of nursing theories and models in nursing researches offers unparalleled contribution to the health care system through the practices of the nurse as a professional. Cultural competence models developed by nurse researchers can be transferred not only to nursing but also to other disciplines.

Leininger describes transcultural nursing as a branch of nursing or nursing school based on comparative research and analysis of different cultures which provides cultural universalism and cultural independence in nursing care and focuses on comparative studies and analyzing differences in cultures around the world in a respectful manner in view of health, illness, care, beliefs and values [3, 5, 13].

The aims of transcultural nursing are to provide sensitive and effective nursing care to meet the cultural needs of individuals, families and groups, to integrate transcultural concepts, theories and practices into nursing education, research and clinical applications, to improve transcultural nursing knowledge, and to incorporate this knowledge into nursing practice.

The International Nurses Association (ICN) invited the nurses from the World Health Organization (WHO) member countries to work on adaptable models to their communities at the 1989 Seoul Conference. The studies conducted in Turkey show that the nurses need to have classification lists and guidelines to be used in care, and thus a more systematic care will be provided in less time for individual patients and more data will be collected. In Turkey internationally developed models and classification systems in nursing care are translated into Turkish, or new guidelines specific to clinics are developed and used. These include NANDA's diagnosis, Gordon's Functional Health Patterns, NIC, NOC and Daily Living Activities and the OMAHA system [55].

The use of transcultural nursing models, classification systems and guidelines is becoming widespread. These models focus on the relationship of nursing to concepts and theories related to life, health, disease and society, facilitate organizing their thoughts, and provide a common language among professional members.

While there has been an increased awareness of the importance of cultural care and collecting cultural data in recent years in Turkey, no models or guides have been developed in Turkey [55].

8.4. Some of these models

8.4.1. Leininger's sunrise model

The "Culture Care Diversity and Universality" theory developed by Leininger in 1960, the first nurse who made the first work in this field and received the title of anthropologist, is the first theory developed in the field of transcultural nursing and still used worldwide. This theory focuses on exploring different and universal cultures and providing comparative care. It adopts a multifactorial approach affecting health and care such as environmental conditions, ethnography, language, gender, class, racism, social structuring, belief, politics, economics, kinship, technology, culture and philosophy. This model includes technological, religious and philosophical, kinship and social factors, cultural values and lifestyle, political and legal, economic and social factors [50], which have been used in many studies in the west and in other countries since 1960 (**Figure 1**).

8.4.2. Narayanasamy's ACCESS model

Narayanasamy described the model in 1998 with the letters ACCESS (Assessment, Communication, Cultural negotiations and Compromise, Establishing respect, Sensitivity and Safety) to form the framework of cultural care practices [42] (**Table 1**).

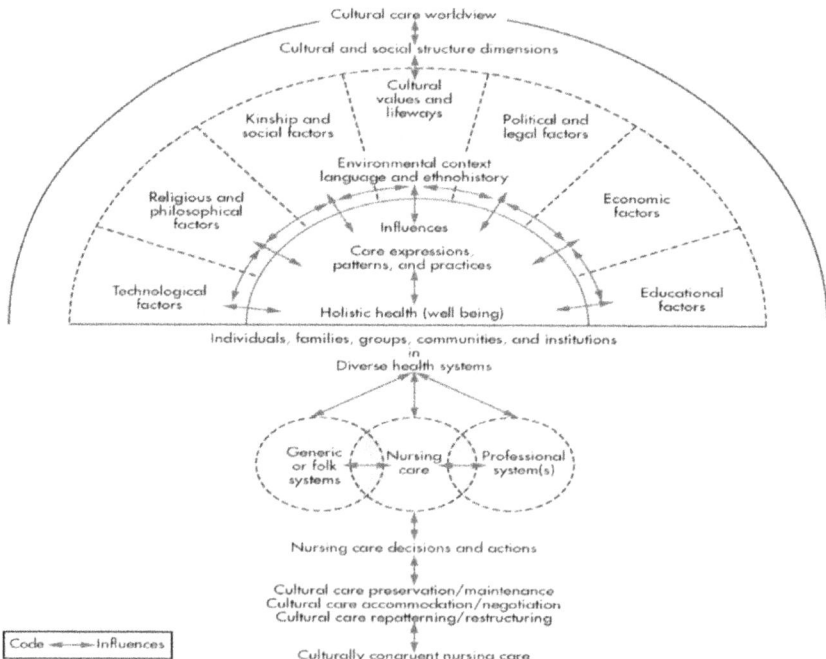

Figure 1. Leininger's sunrise model. Reference: [2].

Transkültürel Hemşirelik	
Assessment	Culturally focusing on the patient's life style, beliefs and practices related to health
Communication	Awareness of the variety of verbal and nonverbal reactions
Cultural Negotiation and Compromise	Becoming more aware of the other people's cultures and exploring their problems as well as understanding the patient's opinion,
Respect	Describing therapeutic relationship relevant to the patient's cultural beliefs and consensus values
Sensitivity	Applying the sensitive care model to culturally different groups
Safety	Making the patient feel safe in the culturally sensitive care
Reference: [2].	

Table 1. Narayanasamy's ACCESS model (1998).

8.4.3. Giger and Davidhizar's transcultural assessment model

The model developed in 1988 was first published in 1990. This model is a tool developed to assess cultural values and their effects on health and disease behavior [33] (**Figure 2**).

8.4.4. Purnell's cultural competence model

This ethnographic model created to promote cultural understanding of people's status in the context of health promotion and illness is based on ethical perspectives of individual, family and community. It can be used in primary, secondary and tertiary protection stages [56] (**Figure 3**).

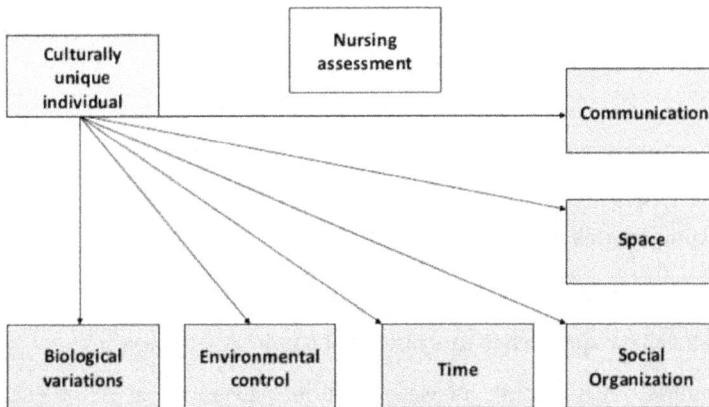

Figure 2. Giger and Davidhizar's transcultural assessment model. Reference: [33].

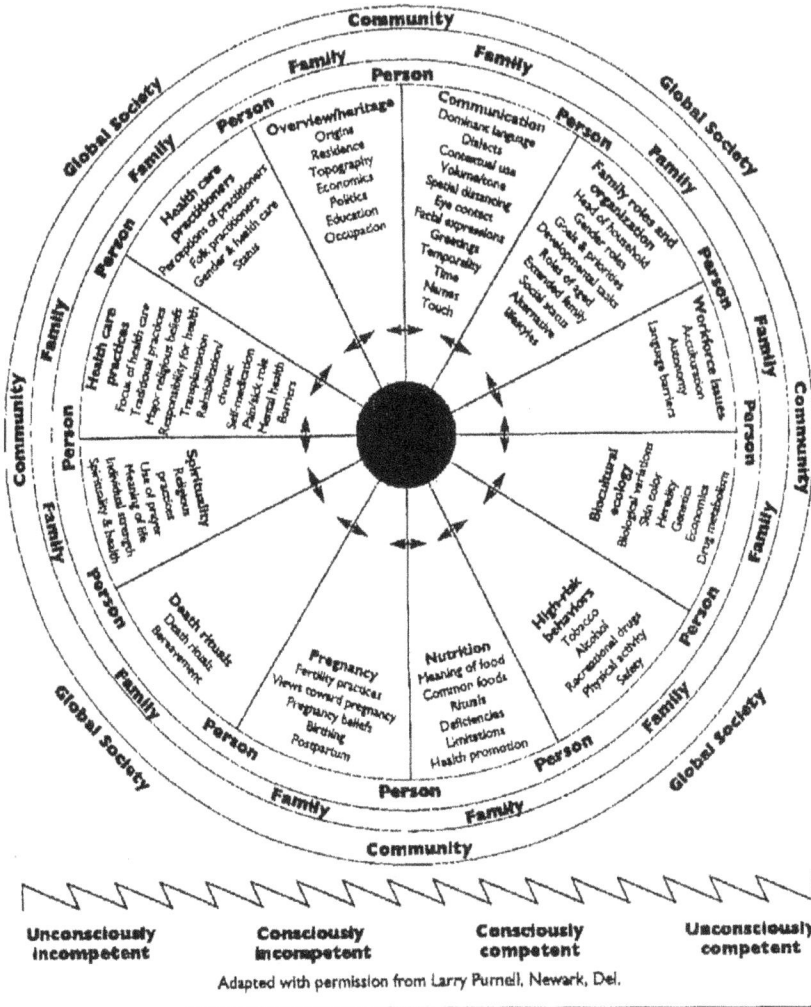

Figure 3. Purnell's model for cultural competence. A care preparation that is accepted as appropriate from a cultural perspective requires that the nurse personally develops, perfects and uses specific skills. Reference: [55].

8.5. Nurses' competences to provide transcultural care

- Having the ability to understand complex cultural dimensions,
- Assuming a holistic approach to care instead of biophysical approach,
- Showing efforts to reach rapidly increasing cultural beliefs and activities that are unique to distinct groups and individuals

- Being able to change the idea of believing that individuals' own race is superior to others,

- Being able to make cultural evaluations,

- Developing communicative and scientific language skills,

- Being able to deal with cultural differences in real terms and make interpretations,

- Being able to use appropriate cultural teaching techniques

- Compromising cultural beliefs and studies with the general state of provision of health care,

- Respecting for the sociocultural diversity of women, newborn babies and their families [8, 57].

9. Transcultural nursing education

The ability of nurses to change their current and future nursing practices through transcultural nursing care approach in the nursing care system can be achieved through cultural specific transcultural nursing education programs [22, 58].

Regardless of their ethnic characteristics, nursing educators have great responsibilities to develop positive attitudes towards intercultural nursing care as a role model for their students [29, 58].

In addition, registered nurses should be aware of these issues and develop their knowledge and competence. Educators and administrators need to know, understand and believe in the importance of intercultural nursing care in order to be role models for students. The first step in the development and implementation of intercultural nursing education programs in nursing institutions is to evaluate the curriculum. It is recommended that the review in nursing schools be started with an examination of the mission statement. It should be examined whether the significance of cultural differences, care and education are explained in the mission statement [58, 59].

The multicultural education approach and educational program should replace the dominant cultures in nursing schools. With the help of this approach, school administrators and academics should observe whether content issues are appropriate and adequate in terms of multicultural education in current educational programs [58].

In terms of multiculturalism, important main subjects, concepts, theories should be defined and integrated into the curriculum [59].

The terms such as cultural competence, multiculturalism, cultural diversity, cultural awareness, cultural safety should be intertwined with other professional subjects into the curriculum.

An educational environment should be created in which racial differences are accepted and respected in nursing education. Within the scope of the program, generalizations and conceptualizations specific to different cultural groups should be introduced in theoretical and practical courses. During the courses social problems, experiences brought about by different racetracks such as racism, prejudicial discrimination, language problems, communicative difficulties, lack of obtaining information, health services that do not meet the needs, lack of recognition or determination of diagnosis, and incorrect nursing diagnosis should be discussed [58–61].

Students can examine and evaluate their racial characteristics in the communication and skills lab. In addition, similarities and differences between ethnic groups should be emphasized in all lectures [58, 59].

In intercultural nursing education, the students' ethnocentric worldview "just like me" should be replaced by the view "not like me". It is stated in the nursing education that it is very useful for the student to assume some duties and responsibilities in community services and health education programs to develop cultural competence [58].

In addition, it has been shown that the exchange of national and international students and teaching staff in nursing schools is a very useful way to build cultural awareness and sensitivity by experiencing, working, and living in another culture, in order for students to find intercultural opportunities in different cultural settings [58, 62, 63].

It is stated that it is a useful teaching method for nurses to teach nursing diagnoses with case studies involving different cultural items in education programs. In nursing programs focusing on intercultural education, nursing educators use methods and tools such as critical reflection, discussion groups, role playing, observations, simulation exercises, clinical scenarios as well as written materials, videos, film monitoring and audio tapes [58].

10. Criticisms of transcultural nursing

Although transcultural nursing has an important role in the holistic approach, it is criticized at some points and is also mentioned in opposing views.

In the case of launching nationalist initiatives in intercultural care, it has been stated that stereotyped images may emerge, and that particular attention may be paid to certain cultural individuals in the caring process. Given the presence of some 3000 cultures around the world, it is impossible for healthcare professionals to have knowledge of all cultures. It also requires the specialization of health personnel in order to provide qualified, culturally specific care. Despite the desire to create multicultural societies in the world in which there are liberal immigrant policies, it cannot be argued that there is an accepted standard in health care, in terms of the socioeconomic status, ethnic characteristics, sexual behavior and lifestyle preferences. There is a cultural crisis in health care services. Individualized intercultural care is a nurse's responsibility as both a human and a professional. However, it is noted that nurses may be ethnocentric with cultural knowledge, understanding, awareness, education, cultural competence and lack of faith [58].

It is argued that extraordinary endeavors in cultural sensitivity can result in the classification of cultures, thereby leading to stereotyped behaviors in certain cultures, races and religions. Another criticism is that paying particular attention to the patient of a particular culture, and focusing on that side can cause limitations in care. It is emphasized that the patient may feel "special", "needing protection" or "patronized". In addition, it has been pointed out that concerns about transcultural care in the field of health will only lead to formation of specialization in transcultural care that could increase responsibilities for nurses, which in turn will put a burden on them [2].

Conflict of interest

The authors declare that they have no conflict of interest.

Funding

No outside funding was received for this study.

Author details

Vasfiye Bayram Değer

Address all correspondence to: vasfiyedeg@gmail.com

School of Health Sciences, Artuklu University, Mardin, Turkey

References

[1] TDK. What is Culture? http://www.tdk.gov.tr/index.php?option=com_gts&kelime=K%C3%9CLT%C3%9CR [Accessed: December 6, 2017]

[2] Hotun Şahin N, Onat Bayram G, Avcı D. Responsive approach to cultures: Transcultural nursing. Journal of Nursing Education and Research. 2009;6(1):2-7

[3] Öztürk E, Öztaş D. Transcultural nursing. Batman University Journal of Life Sciences. 2012;1(1):293-300

[4] İz B, Bayık Temel A. Cultural competence in nursing. Family and Society. 2009;5(17):51-58

[5] Tortumoğlu G. Examples of transcultural nursing and cultural care models. Cumhuriyet University Nursing School Journal. 2004;8(2):47-57

[6] Spradley BW. Community Health Nursing Concepts and Practice. Boston: Little Brown and Company; 1981. pp. 553-569

[7] Degazon C. Community health nursing. In: Stanhope M, Lancaster J, editors. Cultural Diversity and Community Health Nursing Practice. Baltimore: MosbyYearBook; 1996. pp. 117-134

[8]   Bolsoy N, Sevil Ü. Health-disease and culture interaction. Atatürk University Nursing School Journal. 2006;**9**(3):78-87

[9]   Allen J. Improving cross-cultural care and antiracism in nursing education: A literature review. Nurse Education Today. 2010;**30**(4):314-320

[10] Domenig D. Transcultural change: A challenge for the public health system. Applied Nursing Research. 2004;**17**(3):213-216

[11] Yaman Aktaş Y, Gök Uğur H, Orak OS. Investıgatıon of the opinions of nurses concerning the transcultural nursing care. International Refereed Journal of Nursing Researches. 2016;**8**:120-135

[12] Tanrıverdi G, Bayat M, Sevig U, Birkök C. Evaluation of the effect of cultural characteristics on use of health care services using the 'Giger and Davidhizar's transcultural assessment model: A sample from a village in Eastern Turkey. Dokuz Eylül Üniversitesi Hemşirelik Fakültesi Elektronik Dergisi. 2011;**4**:19-24

[13] Tortumoğlu G, Okanlı A, Özer N. Cultural approach and its importance in nursing care. International Journal of Human Sciences. 2004;**10**(2):1-12. ISSN: 1303-5134

[14] Kuğuoğlu S. Transcultural nursing. In: Aslan FE, editor. Internal and Surgical Care Ayfer Karadakovan. Adana: Nobel Kitabevi; 2011. pp. 91-104

[15] Tabak R. Health culture and youth. In: 8th National Public Health Congress; Diyarbakır; 2002. pp. 567-569

[16] Andrews MM, Boyle JS. Transcultural concepts in nursing care. Journal of Transcultural Nursing. 2002;**13**(3):178-180

[17] Boyle JS. Transcultural nursing: Where do we go from here? Journal of Transcultural Nursing. 2000;**11**(1):10-11

[18] Bekâr M. Intercultural (nursing). Society and Physician. 2001;**16**(2):136-141

[19] Papadopoulos I. Health and illness beliefs of Greek Cypriots living in London. Journal of Advanced Nursing. 1999;**29**(5):1097-1104

[20] Uosukainen LM. Promotion of the good life by public health nurses. Public Health Nursing. 2001;**18**(6):375-384

[21] Mattson S. Working toward cultural competence. Making the first steps through cultural assessment. AWHONN Lifelines/Association of Women's Health, Obstetric and Neonatal Nurses. 2000;**4**(4):41-43

[22] Duffy ME. A critique of cultural education in nursing. Journal of Advanced Nursing. 2001;**36**(4):487-495

[23] Papadopoulos I. The Papadopoulos, Tilki and Taylor model for the development of cultural competence in nursing. Journal of Health, Social and Environmental Issues. 2003;**4**:5-7

[24] Serrant-Green L. Transcultural nursing education: A view from within. Nurse Education Today. 2001;**21**(8):670-678

[25] Sivri B, Karataş N. Cultural aspects of society: Traditional practices and examples from the world towards maternal care in the postnatal period. The Journal of Current Pediatrics. 2015;**13**:183-193

[26] Gustafson DL. Transcultural nursing theory from a critical cultural perspective. Advances in Nursing Science. 2005;**28**(1):2-16

[27] Jeffreys MR. Development and psychometric evaluation of the transcultural self-efficacy tool (TSET): A synthesis of findings. Journal of Transcultural Nursing. 2000;**11**(2):127-136

[28] Maıer-Lorentz MM. Transcultural nursing: Its importance in nursing practice. Journal of Cultural Diversity. 2008;**15**(1):37-43

[29] Narayanasamy A, Whıte E. A review of transcultural nursing. Nurse Education Today. 2005;**25**(2):102-111

[30] Leınınger M, Mcfarland M. Transcultural Nursing Concepts, Theories, Research and Practice. Third ed. New York, USA: McGraw-Hill Companies; 2002. pp. 3-44

[31] Kanıtsakı O. Transcultural nursing and challenging the status quo. Contemporary Nurse. 2003;**15**(3):5-9

[32] Leınınger M. Culture care theory: A major contribution to advance transcultural nursing knowledge and practices. Journal of Transcultural Nursing. 2002;**13**(3):189-192

[33] Gıger J, Davidhizar R. The Giger and Davidhizar transcultural assessment model. Journal of Transcultural Nursing. 2002;**13**(3):185-188

[34] Campınha-Bacote J. The process of cultural competence in the delivery of healthcare services: A model of care. Journal of Transcultural Nursing. 2002;**13**(3):181-184

[35] Domenig D. Transcultural change: A challenge for the public health system. Applied Nursing Research. 2004;**17**(3):213-216

[36] Kılıç SP, Besen DB, Tokem Y, Fadıloğlu Ç, Karadağ G. An analysis of the cultural problems encountered during caregiving by the nurses working in two different regions of Turkey. International Journal of Nursing Practice. 2014;**20**(3):310-319

[37] Ayaz S, Bilgili N, Akın B. The transcultural nursing concept: A study of nursing students in Turkey. International Nursing Review. 2010;**57**(4):449-453

[38] Tanrıverdı G, Okanlı A, Şıpkın S, Özyağcılar N, Akyıl R. The evaluation of the cultural differences experienced by nursing and midwifery students in nursing. Dokuz Eylül Üniversitesi Hemşirelik Yüksekokulu Elektronik Dergisi. 2010;**3**(3):117-122

[39] Tortumoğlu G, Okanlı A, Ozyazıcığlu N, Akyıl R. Defining cultural diversities experienced in patient care by nursing students in eastern Turkey. Nurse Education Today. 2006;**26**(2):169-175

[40] Poss JE. Providing culturally competent care: Is there a role for health promoters? Nursing Outlook. 1999;**47**(1):30-36

[41] Engebretson J, Mahoney J, Carlson ED. Cultural competence in the era of evidence-based practice. Journal of Professional Nursing. 2008;**24**(3):172-178

[42] Narayanasamy A. The ACCESS model: A transcultural nursing practice framework. The British Journal of Nursing. 2002;**11**(9):643-650

[43] Higginbottom GM. Heart health-associated health beliefs and behaviours of adolescents of African and African Caribbean descent in two cities in the United Kingdom. Journal of Advanced Nursing. 2000;**32**(5):1234-1242

[44] Flowers DL. Culturally competent nursing care. Critical Care Nurse. 2004;**24**:48-52

[45] Bacote CJ. The process of cultural competence in the delivery of health-care services: A model of care. Journal of Transcultural Nursing 20002;**13**(3):181-184

[46] Eunyoung ES. The model cultural competence through an evolutionary concept analysis. Journal of Transcultural Nursing. 2004;**15**(2):93-110

[47] Zuwang SM. Cultural competence models in nursing: A selected annotated bibliography. Journal of Transcultural Nursing. 2004;**15**(4):317-322

[48] Vydelingum V. Nurses' experiences of caring for South Asian minority ethnic patients in a general hospital in England. Nursing Inquiry. 2006;**13**(1):23-32

[49] Chenowethm L, Jeon YH, Goff M, Burke C. Cultural competency and nursing care: An Australian perspective, International Council of Nurses. International Nursing Review. 2006;**53**:34-40

[50] Leininger MM, McFarland MR. Culture Care Diversity and Universality: A Worldwide Nursing Theory. 2nd ed. Boston: Jones & Bartlett Publishers; 2005

[51] Mattson S. Providing care. The changing face of the US. Lifelines. 2000;**4**(3):49-52

[52] Narayan MC. Cultural assessment in home healthcare. Home Healthcare Nurse. 1997;**15**:663-670

[53] Douglas MK. Standards of practice for culturally competent nursing care. Journal of Transcultural Nursing. 2011;**22**(4):317-333

[54] Ay F. International nursing diagnoses and classification systems used in the field. Turkish Journal of Medical Sciences. 2008:555-561

[55] Tanrıverdi G, Bayat M, Sevig Ü, Birkök MC. Guide to diagnosis of cultural characteristics in nursing care. International Journal of Human Sciences. 2009;**6**(1):793-805

[56] Purnell L. The Purnell model for cultural competence. Journal of Transcultural Nursing. 2002;**13**(3):193-196

[57] Callster LN. Culturally competent care of women and newborns: Knowledge, attitude, and skills. Journal of Obstetric, Gynecologic, and Neonatal Nursing. 2001;**30**:209-215

[58] Bayık TA. Intercultural (multicultural) nursing education. Atatürk University Nursing School Journal. 2008;**11**(2):92-101

[59] White HL. Implementing the multicultural education perspective into the nursing education curriculum. Journal of Instructional Psychology. 2003;**30**(4):326-332

[60] Narayanasamy A. Transcultural nursing: How do nurses respond to cultural needs? British Journal of Nursing. 2003;**12**(2):36-45

[61] Nairn S, Hardy C, Paramal L, et al. Multicultural or anti-racist teaching in nurse education: A critical appraisal. Nurse Education Today. 2004;**24**(3):188-195

[62] Wimpenny P, Goulth B, Mac Lennan V, et al. Teaching and learning about culture: An European journey. Nurse Education Today. 2005;**25**(5):398-404

[63] Koskinen L, Tossavainen K. Characteristics of İntercultural mentoring—A mentor perspective. Nurse Education Today. 2003;**23**(4):278-285

How to Solve Conflicts between Nurses and Patients: Examination from Japanese Culture

Mayumi Uno

Additional information is available at the end of the chapter

http://dx.doi.org/10.5772/intechopen.75936

Abstract

In consideration of the influence of Japanese culture, introduce studies for resolving con-flict between nurses and patients. Japanese have a culture that does not express their thoughts in words. That elegant culture sometimes cannot attract each other's ideas. When it is driven in a busy environment or spiritually, Doi calls it "the structure of amae." However, there seems to be no English equivalent to this *"Amae"*. However, I think that it is very important to understand the concept of *"Amae"* in considering the relationship between a nurse and a patient. Therefore, from the conflict between the nurse and the patient, in particular here we introduce Japanese traditional art "intervention study using tea ceremony: in Japanese *Chadoh"* and "avoidance of veteran nurses conflict". In addi-tion, although these findings are unique to Japan, they can be said to be universal from the viewpoint of human relations.

Keywords: nurse-patient relation, cultural background, conflict

1. Introduction

Based on an abundance of available information, patients select a preferred medical institu-tion, from which they receive medical services doi analyzes Japanese expectations from the perspective of "amae" [1]. The Donabedian [2] framework is often referred to in discussions relating to quality of medical care and patient satisfaction. While a patient has certain fixed goals regarding the completeness of care and restoration of health, satisfaction during the treatment period is, in many cases, influenced by the patient's relationship with nurses.

Patient satisfaction is generally influenced by various factors, including technological elements, interpersonal factors, costs, and the environment. Although the measurement of patient satisfaction in different nursing situations might be complex [3–6], it is generally accepted that patient satisfaction is an important indicator of the quality of the nursing service. Patient satisfaction correlates positively with nursing care and perceptions of the quality of patient service [7]. There is also a strong correlation between satisfaction with nursing care and general satisfaction [8]. Therefore, quality of nursing care, as perceived by patients.

According to Uno et al. [9], patients assume that nurses are bound to utilize appropriate techniques and expressions within the nurse-patient relationship.

In nursing practice, studies by inductive content analysis of cases where conflict has occurred present the conflict situation according to two (2) axes, namely, "impact on the patient" and the "patient's response." The latter suggest that, in the absence of clear patient communication, paying attention to "the effect (of interaction) on the patient's daily mood" is an important sub-service in nursing.

We also compared expectations regarding nursing sub-services, using Parasuraman et al.'s SERVQUAL (Multiple Item Scale for Measuring Consumer Perceptions of Service Quality) [10, 11]. The results showed that patients' expectations of nurses are influenced by the *Omotenashi* culture of "consideration of others," which is characteristic of Japanese people [12].

In an interview with a person who, after serving as a nursing director, still felt it important to be involved with patients [13], we learned that a good nurse deduces the expectations of patients and, interpreting such in terms of nursing science, performs nursing care accordingly. Thus, in this instance, we focused on Gold Nurses or Expert Nurses. To our knowledge, there are no studies focusing on the words (in the form of text) of subjects, to determine aspects of conflict avoidance between nurses and patients. In view of this, we set out to determine this in the specified manner.

In recent years, the clinical practice, education, and research capabilities of nurses have increased; however, there remain complaints from patients and their family members concerning their interactions with nurses. To promote a sense of patient satisfaction during medical treatment, nurses should be aware of subservices that provide insight into the feelings of patients and that facilitate appropriate nurse-patient interactions [14]. Although the goals of nursing include consideration, compassion, and empathy toward patients, there is no concrete method of engendering these in a nurse.

Henderson noted that in the nurse-patient relationship, "getting under his/her skin" is a way to understand a patient [15]. Erikson considered empathy to be "feeling concern for suffering," and showed that a nurse must acknowledge a patient's suffering to make the patient feel they are respected as a person [16]. To alleviate a patient's suffering, a nurse should discover the patient's desires, and the patient's feelings of trust, hope, powerlessness, guilt, and shame [17]. A nurse needs to understand each patient's unique experience of his or her disease, knowledge, and feelings [16, 18]. Such a nurse-patient relationship is considered the foundation of a therapeutic relationship.

Keenan reported that the Japanese tea ceremony is useful for stress management in nurses [19], and Donnelly reported that by placing participants within a natural setting [20], the tea ceremony allows participants to enjoy the life that is universally shared by humans and to maintain harmony with others. Uno reported on the importance of hospitality (in Japanese: *omotenashi*) in the Japanese culture as a characteristic of the nursing interactions that were desired by patients [21]. Although the Japanese tea ceremony is a part of the traditional Japanese culture, few Japanese individuals practice the art daily, and reports concerning the role of the tea ceremony in the field of nursing are rare. Thus, in this study, nurses who worked in a clinical practice participated in the Japanese tea ceremony to evaluate changes in their awareness with respect to their interactions with patients. I focused on the Japanese tea ceremony as a method to form peaceful interpersonal relationships during patient interactions.

2. Conflict occurring between nurse and patient

2.1. Nurse - patient relationship and conflict

High-quality nursing is based on good nurse-patient relationships. Watson described that this relationship is dependent on the nurse's ability to be genuine, authentic, and open [22]. Conventionally, one of the main concepts in nurse-patient relationships is empathy. The concept of "empathy" on the part of nurses replaced the previous concept of "sympathy," which was advocated by Nightingale. For nurses to provide quality care, one researcher advocated that "the nurse must always be kind and sympathetic, but never emotional" [23]. Sympathy in the nurse-patient relationship was recognized as being helpful during the therapeutic process [24, 25]. Henderson described "getting under his/her skin" as a method for nurses to better understand patients [15]. Bissell et al. suggested that good nurse-patient relationships were maintained by building mutual understanding, and described that conflict might arise when this did not occur [26]. Robbins defined conflict as "a process which starts when an individual recognizes that an important matter to him/her was, or would be, adversely affected by another individual," and described that the common point of the definition of conflict in various researchers was "opposition" or "disagreement." Robbins also suggested that conflict exists in four stages. Specifically, these stages are (1) potential opposition, (2) recognition and individualization, (3) behavior, and (4) result [27]. Unoet al. examined conflict that occurred between nurses and patients and reported that recognizing subtle changes patient's feelings might improve nursing [28]. Furthermore, Uno emphasized that what patients expected most during conflict was the concept of empathy, specifically in terms of empathy being defined as the inference of feelings [29]. It was then proposed by Uno et al. that expert nurses would be more likely to exhibit sufficient levels of empathy and revealed that these individuals avoided conflict by guarding the patient's soul and committing to it deeply, while simultaneously keeping appropriate distance [30].

In a study focusing on the circumstances leading to conflict between nurses and patients that was performed by Uno et al. nurse perceptions of patient's expectations under conflict were analyzed both qualitatively and inductively [31]. A total of five categories were extracted: Inference, Empathic understanding, Listening, Individual treatment, and Reliable skills and explanations. Specifically, it was reported that Inference was abnormal in Japanese culture. Thus, it seems that such patient expectations may influence the quality of nursing perceived by patients.

2.2. Understanding of the phenomenon within the clinical setting

Interviews are one method to search for unclear issues within qualitative studies. In an interview, questions and responses exist coincidentally, and the response reflects each interviewee's subjective feeling or thoughts at that time. Conversely, in a descriptive questionnaire survey, as compared to an interview, the response is obtained from subjects after sufficient recollection, which achieves more objective data.

It is difficult to quantify phenomena in clinical settings where nurses face patients. Patient's informal expression of symptoms, such as onomatopoeia (i.e., "*zukizuki*" (describes headache), which is commonly used in clinical settings, can be understood by nurses with experience. In other words, nurses understand and address the phenomenon (patient's complaint) as it deviates from the concept.

3. Compassion for others based on Japanese culture

3.1. "Doh" or "OMOTENASHI" symbolizing Japanese culture

There is Doh" as a traditional technique in Japan. Typical examples are Japanese tea ceremony, flower arrangement, calligraphy and so on.

There is a "hospitality (in Japanese OMOTENASHI)" that treats you with a flexible attitude.

3.2. Japanese tea ceremony

This study provided foundational data for use in nursing interventional methods for improving nurse-patient relationships. This was a descriptive study on the effectiveness of a Japanese tea ceremony (in Japanese: *chado*) intervention for improving nurse-patient relationships. I conducted a Japanese tea ceremony and examined changes in nurses' awareness regarding interactions with patients after this intervention. The tea ceremonies were conducted with the cooperation of an *Urasenke* tea ceremony lecturer. A quiet environment with chairs and tables was provided for all participants while they provided written answers to a descriptive survey, which was administered before and after the intervention; they required approximately 20 min to complete the survey. The mean length of each nurse's description was 800 characters. The tea ceremony was effective in bringing about definite changes in nurses' awareness concerning interactions with patients. This study is useful in that it suggests how nurses can maintain good interpersonal relationships with patients.

This study provided basic data to explore interventional methods for nurses to improve nurse-patient relationships. I examined the manner in which awareness of the nurses regarding their patient interactions changed after participating in the Japanese tea ceremony.

3.3. How to arrange the minds of nurses; introduce a study about to use Japanese tea ceremony

3.3.1. Methods

This study was a descriptive survey of a Japanese tea ceremony intervention. In 2014, I conducted a similar intervention involving three participants and descriptive surveys, similar to those used in the present study. I confirmed that there were no mental or physical burdens on the participants and that there was a change in nurses' awareness.

3.3.2. Participants

I initially mailed 100 regional medical care support hospitals in the Kinki region of Japan to explain the purpose and methods of the study and to request their cooperation. Four hospitals agreed to cooperate. A total of 14 nurses expressed an interest in participating in the present study; however, only 12 nurses were included for analysis because two dropped out during the study. Twelve was the maximum number of individuals who agreed to cooperate. However, the 800 words provided in total by these individuals were sufficient for qualitative summarization.

3.3.3. Data collection

The study period was from March to May 2015. Interventions were performed once per week over a 4-week period (i.e., a total of four times). Interventions were performed in a tea ceremony room located in a temple in the Osaka Prefecture, Japan.

3.3.4. Operational definitions of the terminology

The "Japanese tea ceremony" (in Japanese: *chado*) is a traditional Japanese art that has been referred to as a "composite art form." "Tactfulness in silence" refers to the insight of sensing the thoughts and feelings of others that are not expressed in words.

3.3.5. Study design

I administered a pre-intervention survey to assess the individual characteristics of the nurses (age, years of experience as a nurse, affiliated hospital wards, and experience participating in tea ceremonies) and the following items:

A. Interactions with nurses believed to be desired by patients,

B. Awareness of daily interactions with patients,

C. Interactions believed to improve the quality of nursing, and

D. Image of the tea ceremony.

A quiet environment with chairs and tables was provided for the participants while they provided written answers to the survey.

The tea ceremonies were conducted with the cooperation of an *Urasenke* tea ceremony lecturer. The tea ceremony lecturer acted as the tea master during the ceremonies.

The guests were the participants, who were divided into groups of six individuals; each experienced the same program content for approximately 1 h in each session. To ease the tension of the participants who were participating in the tea ceremony for the first time, the researchers, who had participated in a tea ceremony before, presented a partial example of a ceremony. However, to avoid influencing the study results, the participants were allowed to act naturally during the tea ceremony (**Figures 1** and **2**). The tea ceremony steps are listed below.

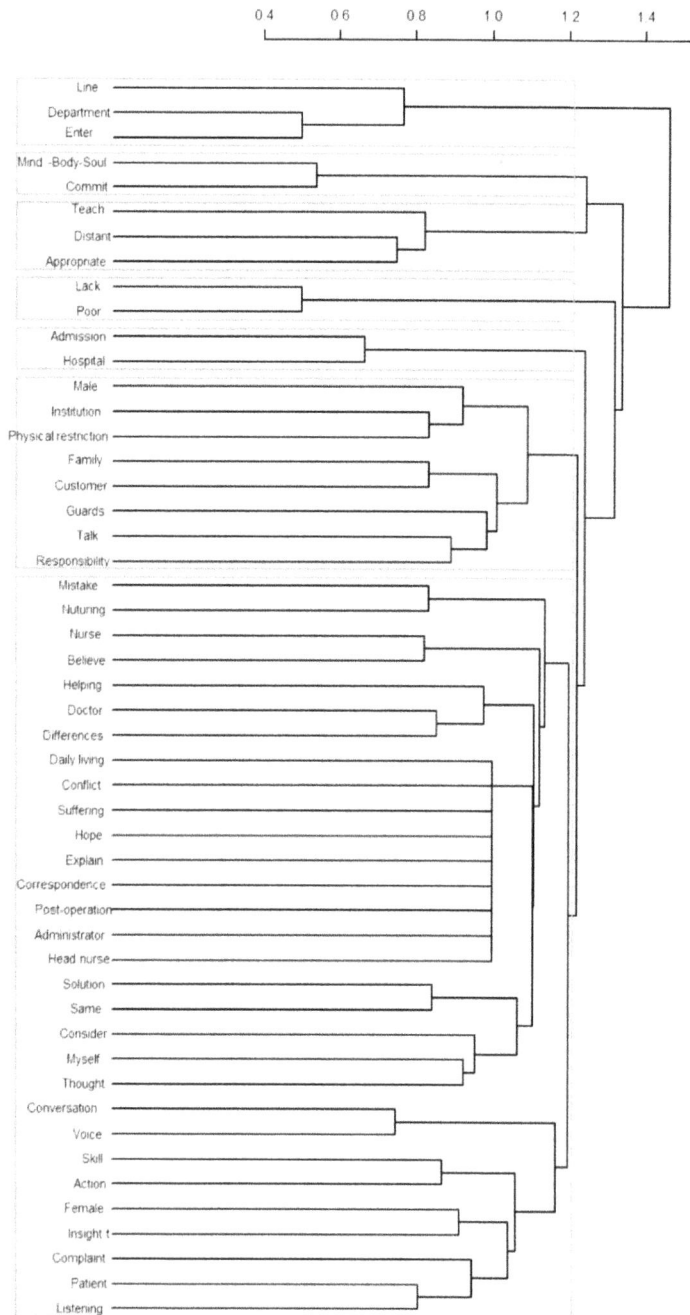

Figure 1. Cluster analysis where gold nurses avoid conflicts.

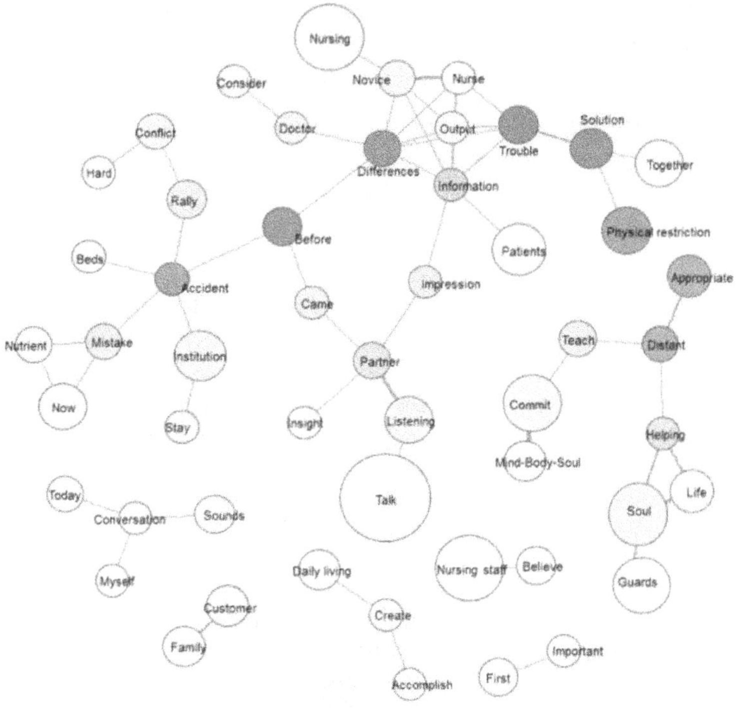

Figure 2. Co-occurrence network analysis where gold nurses avoid conflicts.

3.4. Results

3.4.1. Individual characteristics

The mean age of the 12 participants, all of whom were female, was 48 years (SD = 6.6). The mean years of nursing experience was 23 (SD = 5.8). The nurses worked in the Department of Internal Medicine (chronic disease ward), and no participants had previous experience participating in a tea ceremony. Four of the nurses qualified at a university and eight were qualified as nurses at a vocational school.

3.4.2. Nurse's consciousness of interactions with patients before and after intervention

The participants required approximately 20 min to write their descriptions. The mean length of each nurse's description was 800 characters. The descriptions of items A through D were qualitatively analyzed and compared before and after the intervention

A. **Interactions nurses believed to be desired by patients.** Prior to the intervention the interactions desired were thought to be smiling, kindness, communication, providing explanations, and so forth. After the intervention, the desired interactions were considered to be not superficial gentleness, but rather treating the patient as a person. Patients were believed to expect nurses to stare at them deeply, as it could help them in realizing who that patient is.

B. **Awareness of daily interactions with patients**. Before the intervention points raised were interacting gently and kindly, interacting safely, providing science-based explanations and having a science-based skillset, and displaying an empathetic attitude. After the intervention, the goal was to interact without pressure, such as by providing appropriate space (distance) for the patient.

C. **Interactions believed to improve the quality of nursing.** Before the intervention, the issues raised were to keep learning, learn and practice ways of communicating regarding disease, always think about the patient's feelings, do not make medical mistakes, and so forth; essentially, to provide a good recuperative environment. After the intervention, the participants raised the points: Always tell yourself to be casual (which was helpful for easing their tension), and to "catch precisely, as soon as possible." Furthermore, touch according to the patient's desire. In this way, the participants were transformed such that they could recognize their natural involvement as a person before their involvement as a nurse.

D. **Image of tea ceremony.** Prior to the intervention, the ceremony was considered stiff, difficult, and unfamiliar; only something that rich people learn. After the intervention, it transformed into something that the participants felt they could incorporate into daily life. It was noted that "my own heart calms down."

3.5. Discussion

Results of the pre-intervention awareness analysis revealed an awareness of appropriate professional interactions, such as "interacting gently and kindly," "interacting safely," "explanations and skills with a scientific basis," and "empathetic attitude." The Japanese tea ceremony involves silent communication between the host and guests, as the guests "sensitively feel the intentions of the tea master, who takes great pains to provide an atmosphere of hospitality." The post-intervention comments were related to peaceful interactions, such as "interacting without pressure," "interacting while maintaining an appropriate distance," "interacting with a sincere attitude," and "insight in sensing feelings that are not expressed in words." These categories were based on an awareness of the interactions with patients that were not limited to their status as a professional nurse.

Considering three aspects, I assessed how participant's awareness changed regarding interactions with patients after the tea ceremony. The first aspect was related to changes in feelings because of being in a teahouse and the formal interpersonal relationships that were created. After the intervention, categories related to calmness of mind were suggested by the nurses. For the nurses who were busy with daily nursing tasks, the Japanese tea ceremony was a place where they could relax and find peace of mind. The second aspect was that the participants (nurses) received polite hospitality and were cared for. People tend to be rude to others when they are treated rudely themselves. The work of nurses constitutes emotional labor, that is, the management of emotions in the workplace [9]. After the intervention, the categories "interacting with a sincere attitude" and "insight in sensing feelings that are not expressed in words" were observed. Therefore, the tea ceremony is useful for controlling emotions through polite hospitality and caring for guests.

The third aspect was the way in which the five senses were utilized. Nurses should have a high degree of sensitivity while working in a hectic and highly stressful environment. However, here the participants were given a chance to return to nature by appreciating seasonal flowers. That is, the participants were able to relax in a beautiful environment that could be experienced through the five senses. These findings are important for managing the working environment of nurses, who are likely busy with numerous other daily tasks when interacting with patients.

The program used in this study exceeded the limits of the field of nursing, but it appeared useful for creating favorable nurse-patient relationships. Specifically, this method effectively relaxed the nurses, which suggests that relaxation is one way to improve interpersonal relationships. In summary, the intervention method used in this study is useful for nurses to maintain good interpersonal relationships with patients.

3.6. Conclusions

Changes in nurses' awareness related to interactions with patients were noted after the tea ceremony intervention. I observed changes related to increased functional beauty and spirituality, as exemplified by the categories "interacting without pressure," "interacting while maintaining an appropriate distance," "interacting with a sincere attitude," and "insight in sensing feelings that are not expressed in words." Thus, participating in the tea ceremony was effective in bringing about definite changes in nurses' awareness concerning interactions with patients. However, a future study with an increased sample size is needed to verify the present study's results, and a survey of patients who received nursing care from the participants is also necessary.

4. How to arrange the minds of nurses; introduce a study about aspects of avoidance of conflict between nurses and patients, according to gold nurses, expert or veteran nurses: A program for raising the quality of nursing

4.1. Aim

The purpose of our study was to ascertain, via language (text), methods of avoiding conflict that could have an impact on the quality of the nursing provided by nurses to patients, with a special focus on Gold Nurses (or Expert Nurses).

4.2. Operational definitions

"Gold Nurses": Nursing professionals who have served as, for example, managers of clinical nurses, public health nurses, and so forth, who continue to work as nursing professionals after retirement, upon registration with the Osaka Municipal Government nursing professional organization. No other prefectures in Japan use this specific term. This term is used to distinguish such nurses from "Expert Nurses," who are still employed (i.e., not yet retired).

4.3. Methods

4.3.1. Subjects

Subjects were five persons registered as "Gold Nurses" with the Japan Nursing Association. Data collection was performed in May 2015, a time that suited the schedule of the Regional Public Health Division. Semi-structured interviews were conducted with the subjects, based on an interview guide. The mean interview time was approximately 50 min per person. After obtaining consent from the subjects, the interviews were recorded using an IC (integrated circuit) recorder.

The interview guide, which was based on Robbins's conflict processes, was concerned with the settings and situations (including latent elements) of conflict occurrence within clinical practice, ways of responding to and avoiding conflict, and methods of handling conflict [27].

4.3.2. Data analysis

The interview contents were transcribed verbatim, and morphological analysis was conducted on the textual data. To ensure that there were no discrepancies in meanings, the words were ordered and a dictionary was created; thereafter, using IBM SPSS Text Analytics for Surveys 4.0.1, the data were analyzed with Statics ver. 22, R ver. 3.1.3.

To ensure accuracy during the analysis process, we were supervised by a university professor who is an expert in text mining.

4.3.3. Ethical considerations

Prior to the interviews, a briefing meeting was held with the subjects, where the aspects of the study were explained verbally and in writing; interviews were conducted with subjects who consented to participate, with the guarantee that the said consent could be withdrawn at any time, without any penalties. The ethics committee at the researcher's affiliate institution (Consent Number 1) granted approval for the commission of the study.

4.4. Results

4.4.1. Demographic characteristics

All the participants were female, with a mean age of 63.5 ± 0.48 years, and mean work experience of 40.5 ± 0.38 years as nurses

4.4.2. Data analysis

4.4.2.1. Frequency analysis

Frequency analysis is the frequency of the appearance of words in morphological analysis. The top five words in order of frequency, from 1 to 5, were "Nurse," "Patient," "Care," "Guard," and "Soul."

4.4.2.2. Cluster analysis

"Cluster analysis" comprises a variety of mathematical methods, used to identify similar items in a dataset.

In this instance, distance between items was determined using the Jaccard method and, on the basis of the dissimilarities found, clustering was performed using Ward's method. The numbers in the upper portion of **Figure 1** show the bond distance between the clusters.

It should be noted that the greater the similarity between clusters, the smaller the number indicating distance, thus, one can see the unique closeness of the clusters, "Mind-Body-Soul · Commit" and "Distant · Appropriate." (**Figure 1** Cluster analysis where gold nurses avoid conflicts).

4.4.2.3. Co-occurrence network analysis

Our fundamental network analysis is one widely used in various fields, including sociology and communication networks, and is based on the mathematical graph theory; as shown in the figure. It comprises V: Vertex (vertices), depicted in the form of a circle, and E: Edge (edges), depicted as a line.

Specifically, expressed words that were in a co-occurrence relation are shown as lines, the size of the circle shows appearance frequency, and the thickness of the line shows the relative strength or weakness of the co-occurrence. In this figure, the darker the color, the greater the emphasis. In addition, the separate figure shows the characteristics of co-occurring words.

In relation to "Bed · Accidents," one can identify concern regarding an accident involving falling from a bed. "Consider · Doctor · Differences" a concept that differs from "medical doctor." The cluster, "Trouble · Solution · Physical Restriction · Together," indicates nurses wondering whether physical restriction (restraint) of patients would lead to the resolution of problems. "Nursing · Novice · Nurse · Output · Trouble" indicates problems that could occur in relation to novice nurses. "Appropriate · Distant" and "Customer · Family" show the nurse maintaining an appropriate distance from the patient and his/her family. "Commit · Mind-Body-Soul" clearly shows a commitment to both the physical and mental aspects of patients. "Helping · Soul · Life · Guards" means that assistance in the patient's life constitutes "guarding" (protecting) the soul, or does it perhaps mean that if one's life is under guard, then it follows that the soul is also under guard? In "Daily Living · Create · Accomplish," we learn that there is "creation" of daily life. "Nursing staff · Believe" indicates that the Expert Nurse has trust in her staff (**Figure 2** Co-occurrence network analysis where gold nurses avoid conflicts).

4.4.3. Excerpts from the text (language) data

A. As a foundation for securing nursing quality, the avoidance of an accident in a nursing situation is most important. Such a situation causes mental discord within a nurse. Although it is possible to restrain a patient, so as to prevent injury to the patient or to prevent an accident, can one really guard a patient and his or her family's soul?

B. We, nurses, are proud to be guarding the souls of our patients.

C. Doctors protect (guard) life as their first priority. We, nurses, protect (guard) the soul as well as the body.

D. The most prominent concern in the mind of a novice nurse is to avoid causing an accident; she (he) might even, at times, forget that the patient is a person. However, that would cause problems between the nurse and the patient, or the patient's family. Yet, I still carry on with my work, while trusting novice nurses and our staff.

E. We are deeply committed to our patients. Meanwhile, we discern aspects within our patients and their lives that we should not delve into.

4.5. Discussion

Nurses have an awareness relating to the question, "What can I do, as a nurse?" (or, "What can we do, as nurses?"). The authors believe that it is precisely such dedicated thinking that raises nursing quality. The Gold Nurses in our study each have very substantial experience working as nurses. The amount of experience in this regard not only shows an accumulation of years, but also indicates refinement of the nurses' theories and conceptualizations, as a result of facing numerous actual situations [32].

The concrete meaning of "guarding the patient's soul" is the fact that the nurse continues to provide care, from the emergency (acute) period through to social rehabilitation; in other words, a nurse's pride is the fact that she (or he) never saves only a life, even in emergency situations. Further, the fact that nurses are deeply committed to their patients indicates insights about their consideration of others, from feelings cultivated during training, to their working together with patients and their families, so as to create and nurture everyday lives, while also recognizing areas that a nurse should not delve into. On this basis, these nurses can avoid conflict in their relationships with patients and families.

Research on customer satisfaction is quite established in business management studies; SERVQUAL is a popular scale for measuring the gap between expectations of general services and customer satisfaction. The five service dimensions comprising this concept are identified as Reliability, Tangibles, Responsiveness, Assurance, and Empathy [33, 34]. Meanwhile, in a study focusing on nurses, Koerner states that, while the conceptual zones of service quality are clarified in Parasuraman et al. [35]., these are not completely accurate for nursing services provided to inpatients. Rather, Compassion, Individual Care, Close Relationships, Uncertainty Reduction, and Reliability are appropriate for the latter instance. Beltrán went on to state the following: "The interaction between patients and nurses goes through various stages until achieving the necessary empathy, compassion, affection, and familiarity to account for humanized care [36]."

In our study, Guarding the Soul, Deep Commitment, and Determining an Appropriate Distance from Patients, were cited as important elements in the configuration of nursing services, the type that Gold Nurses are especially proud of. Although there are reports concerning "Spiritual Care," a concept with a meaning similar to that of Guarding the Soul [37, 38], with regard to the idea that "life" includes the "soul" of the patient in the nurse-patient relationship, we found the following quote by Cumbie to be especially relevant: "Reflected self-awareness is the key to perception of self within the context of human experience." [39]

4.6. Conclusion

Gold Nurses (or Expert Nurses) guard their patients' souls, and while deeply committed, they maintain an appropriate distance, thus, avoiding conflict with patients and enhancing the quality of nursing.

4.7. Relevance to clinical practice

The methods that Gold Nurses (or Expert Nurses) have devised to interact with, and give satisfaction to their patients, raise the quality of nursing. Such can serve as references for novice nurses still worrying about their relationships with patients, in that, if training is provided in such methods, then nurses would be able to gain such valuable experience without having to rely on working as a nurse for many years.

4.8. Limitations

A limitation of our study was the fact that we investigated only the perspectives of nursing service providers. In future, there will be a need to consider issues relating to nursing services from patients' perspective, as well. I appreciate those concerned who cooperated until the completion of the author. To consider nursing service from the Japanese culture. This idea represents the characteristics of interpersonal culture of the Japanese. At the root of the research, we think that the human relationship between nurses and patients is universal.

Acknowledgements

I deeply appreciate my friends who supported me.

Conflict of interest

There is no conflict of interest concerning this writing.

Funding

None.

Author details

Mayumi Uno

Address all correspondence to: unomayu@gmail.com

Graduate School of Medicine, Course of Health Science, Osaka University, Osaka, Japan

References

[1] Doi T. Amae no Kouzou. Kouubndoh. 2014. p. 30-31

[2] Donabedian A. Evaluating the quality of medical care. The Milbank Memorial Fund Quarterly. 1996;**44**:166-206

[3] Zahr LK, William SG, El-Hadad A. Patient satisfaction with nursing care in Alexandria, Egypt. Journal of Nursing Studies. 1991;**28**:337-342

[4] Avis M, Bond M. Satisfying solutions: A review of some unresolved issues in the measurement of patient satisfaction. Journal of Advanced Nursing. 1995;**22**:316-322

[5] Chang K. Dimensions and indicators of patients' perceived nursing care quality in the hospital setting. Journal of Nursing Care Quality. 1977;**11**:26-37

[6] O'Connell B, Young J, Twigg D. Patient satisfaction with nursing care: A measurement conundrum. International Journal of Nursing Practice. 1999;**5**:72-77

[7] Neidz BA. Correlates of hospitalized patients' perceptions of service quality. Research in Nursing & Health. 1988;**21**:339-349

[8] Beck KL, Larrabee JH. Measuring patients' perception of nursing care. Nursing Management. 1996;**27**:32-34

[9] Uno M, Tsujimoto T, Inoue T. Effect of conflicts in patient-nurse relations. Nursing Journal of Osaka University. 2014;**20**(1):47-53

[10] Parasuraman A, Zeithaml V, Berry L, et al. Journal of Marketing. 1985;**49-Fall**:41-50

[11] Parasuraman A, Zeithaml V, Berry L. A multiple-item scale for measuring consumer perceptions of service quality. Journal of Retailing. 1988;**64**(1):12-40

[12] Uno M. A study using Servqual to evaluate trends in patient expectations when conflict arises. Journal of Yamato University. 2014;**1**:173-179

[13] Uno M. Nursing practice: Nursing director of retirement still involved as a staff nurse and patient. The Science of Nursing Practice. 2013;**38**(3):66-69

[14] Uno M, Tsujimoto T, Inoue T. Effect of conflicts in patient-nurse relations. Nursing Journal Osaka University. 2014;**20**:47-53 [in Japanese]

[15] Henderson V. The nature of nursing. American Journal of Nursing. 1964;**64**:62-68

[16] Eriksson K. Understanding the world of the patient, the suffering human beings: The new clinical paradigm from nursing to caring. Advanced Practice Nursing Quarterly. 1997;**3**:8-13

[17] Erikson K. Caring, spirituality and suffering. In: Roach MS, editor. Caring from the Heart: The Convergence of Caring and Spirituality. Mahwah, NJ: Paulist Press; 1997. p. 81

[18] Beech P, Norman IJ. Patients' perception of the quality of psychiatric nursing care: Findings from a small-scale descriptive study. Journal of Clinical Nursing. 1995;**4**:117-123. DOI: 10.1111/j.1365-2702.1995.tb00019.x

[19] Keenan J. The Japanese tea ceremony and stress management. Holistic Nursing Practice. 1996;**10**:30-37

[20] Donnelly GF. The tea ceremony: Connecting with self and others. Holistic Nursing Practice. 2007;**21**:215

[21] Uno M. A study using Servqual to evaluate trends in patient expectations when conflict arises. Journal of Yamato University. 2015;**1**:173-179

[22] Watson J. Nursing: The philosophy and science of caring. Nursing Administration Quarterly. 1979;**3**(4):86-87

[23] Seymer L. Selected Writings of Florence Nightingale. New York, NY: Macmillan; 1954

[24] Orlando IJ. The Dynamic Nurse Patient Relationship. New York: G. P. Putnam; 1961

[25] Peplau HE. Interpersonal Relationships in Nursing. G.P. Putnam: New York, NY; 1952

[26] Bissell P, May C, Noyce PR. From compliance to concordance: Barriers to accomplishing a re-framed model of health care interactions. Social Science & Medicine. 2004;**58**(4):851-862

[27] Robbins SP. Organizational Behavior. 8th ed. Tokyo: Diamond; 2009 [in Japanese]

[28] Uno M, Tsujimoto T, Inoue T. Effect of conflicts in patient-nurse relations. Nursing Journal of Osaka University. 2014;**20**(1):47-53 [in Japanese]

[29] Uno M. A study using Servqual to evaluate trends in patient expectations when conflict arises. Journal of Yamato University. 2015;**1**:173-179

[30] Uno M, Ikuta S, Okamoto M. Aspects of avoidance of conflict between nurses and patients, according to gold nurses (or expert nurses): A program for raising the quality of nursing. Journal of Yamato University. 2016;**2**:91-97

[31] Uno M, Tsujimoto T, Inoue T. Perceptions of nurses in Japan toward their patients' expectations of care: A qualitative study. International Journal of Nursing Sciences. 2017;**4**: 58-62. DOI: 10.1016/j.ijnss.2016.12.005

[32] Benner, Wrubel, Benner P, Wrubel J. Clinical knowledge development: The value of perceptual awareness. Nurse Educator. 1982;**7**:11-17

[33] Parasuraman A, Zeithaml V, Berry L. A conceptual model of service quality and its implications for future research. Journal of Marketing. 1985;**49-Fall**:41-50

[34] Parasuraman A, Zeithaml V, Berry L. A multiple-item scale for measuring consumer perceptions of service quality. Journal of Retailing. 1988;**64**(1):12-40

[35] Korner MM. The conceptual domain of service quality for inpatients nursing services. Journal of Business Research. 2000;**48**:267-283

[36] Beltrán Salazar OA. Humanized care: A relationship of familiarity and affectivity. Investigación y Educación en Enfermenia. 2015;**33**(1):17-27

[37] Bldacchino DR, Draper P. Spiritual coping strategies: A review of the nursing research literature. Journal of Advanced Nursing. 2005;**34**:833-841

[38] Giske T, Cone PH. Discerning the healing path how nurses assist patient spirituality in diverse health care settings. Journal of Clinical Nursing. 2015;**2**:1-10

[39] Cumbie SA. The integration of mind-body-soul and the practice of humanistic nursing. Holistic Nursing Practice. 2001;**15**(3):56-62

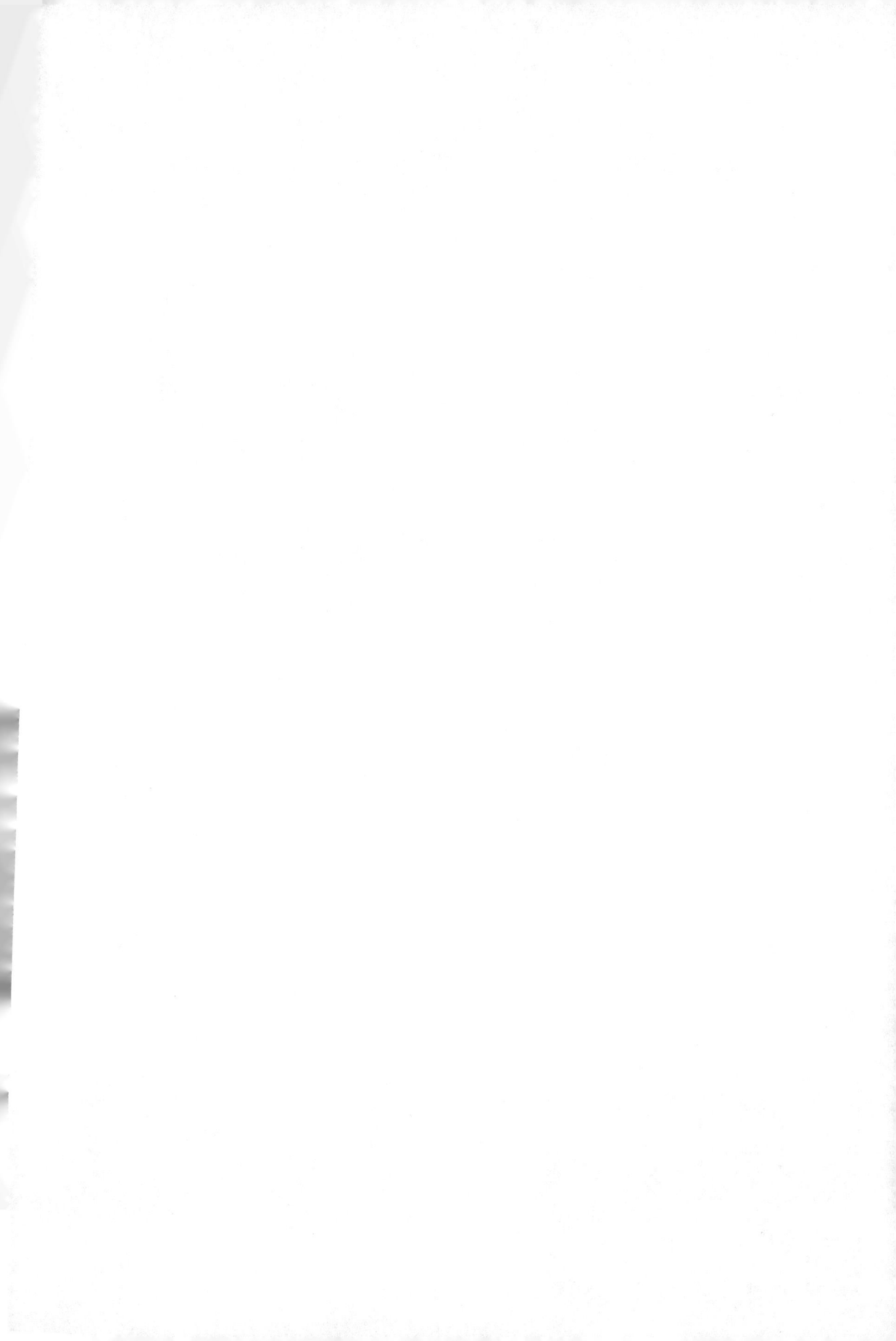